Breaking the Headache Cycle

Breaking
the
Headache
Cycle

◆ A Proven Program
for Treating and Preventing
Recurring Headaches

IAN LIVINGSTONE, M.D.,
and DONNA NOVAK, R.N., M.S.N., N.P.C.

An Owl Book

Henry Holt and Company | New York

Owl Books
Henry Holt and Company, LLC
Publishers since 1866
175 Fifth Avenue
New York, New York 10010
www.henryholt.com

An Owl Book® and 🛡® are registered trademarks
of Henry Holt and Company, LLC.

Library of Congress Cataloging-in-Publication Data

Livingstone, Ian.
    Breaking the headache cycle : a proven program
for treating and preventing recurring headaches /
Ian Livingstone and Donna Novak—1st ed.
        p. cm.
    Includes bibliographical references and index.
    ISBN-13: 978-0-8050-7221-1
    ISBN-10: 0-8050-7221-7
    1. Headache—Popular works. 2. Migraine—
Popular works. I. Novak, Donna. II. Title.

RC392.L585 2003
616.8'4912—dc22   2003056601

Henry Holt books are available for special promotions
and premiums. For details contact: Director, Special Markets.

First Edition 2003

Designed by Victoria Hartman

Printed in the United States of America
10 9 8 7 6 5 4

Dedicated to all migraine sufferers
and to our patients from whom
we have learned so much

Contents

Breaking the Headache Cycle

PART I

Headaches, Stress, and the Nervous System

A Neurologist's Quest
to Treat His Own Migraine:
Dr. Livingstone's Story

I remember my first migraine as vividly as if it occurred yester-day. I was a second-year medical student. The morning following an important anatomy test, I woke up at 4 A.M. with a pounding headache. Light, even from the bedside lamp, was blinding. Sound from the rustling of the sheets was irritating. I could find no comfort as waves of nausea swept through my body. I couldn't decide whether the nausea arose from my stomach or my head. I held my head in my hands, placed a cold cloth on my forehead, and took a painkiller without relief. Any movement worsened the pain. After hours of misery I eventually fell asleep and later awoke with some relief and the feeling that I would survive. "It's just stress," I thought, and this analysis was confirmed by my fel-low medical students, family, and family doctor.

Only years later, during my neurology residency, did I realize that these headaches were migraines, and only recently have I come to understand their relationship to stress.

Several years ago, my headaches became more frequent and more frustrating. Although I love my work, it is stressful. I often skipped meals, kept irregular hours, had interrupted nights, and did not tend to my own well-being. In short, I did not practice what I preached to my patients.

I felt angry and frustrated by my inability to prevent these headaches and increasingly resented the need to take medication in order to function. I also felt cheated because the headaches would often occur on weekends when I was most relaxed. I found myself nursing a headache when I could have been enjoying time with friends and family, and my lack of control over these headaches frustrated me. I knew I needed to look at my own life, to take stock, but I felt enormous resistance to doing so.

I consulted a colleague who suggested I take preventive daily medications. I resisted, thinking that there had to be a more natural way to control these headaches.

I began studying the early medical writings on headache as well as the current scientific literature, looking for a thread that explains our sensitivity to headache and why we are prone to different and diverse headache triggers. I attended seminars. I kept a headache diary. I began listening more closely to my patients. I read Oliver Sacks's *Migraine,* with its poetic description of migraine sufferers. I then came across a monograph written by a Victorian neurologist named Edward Liveing in 1873 entitled *On Megrim, Sick-Headache and Some Allied Disorders: A Contribution to the Pathology of Nerve-Storms.* He wrote this book at a time when there was very little scientific information on headache—at a time when most headaches were considered neurotic in origin. It was a groundbreaking work describing in detail the case histories of numerous migraine sufferers with common patterns. He was the first person to describe the heightened reactivity of the nervous system as part of the migraine trait. We headache sufferers react vigorously to change. This includes sensitivity to stress, sensory overload, odors, certain foods, weather changes, changes in routine, and insufficient sleep or even too much sleep.

Liveing also recognized that migraine is not just a headache but a whole constellation of symptoms of which the head pain is only part. He referred to these as "nerve storms." He had no scientific way to understand that he was observing the effects of fluctuating brain chemistry that occurs with migraine. He was aware of the fact that the tendency of headaches often runs in families, yet he lived more than a hundred years before the discovery of the DNA genetic coding of the first migraine genes.

As I followed this theory of sensitivity through old and modern medical writings I was led back to one of my main passions in studying neurology—the relationship of mind and body.

The Natural Way to Reduce Headache

I wondered if there were natural and scientifically based ways to calm and protect the sensitivity of the nervous system. And if so, do these techniques improve the quality of life of those who suffer recurring headache?

The answers came when I attended one of Dr. Herbert Benson's seminars. Dr. Benson, the discoverer of the "relaxation response," is founding president of the Mind/Body Medical Institute at the Beth Israel Deaconess Medical Center. I began to look for ways to tailor relaxation techniques to headache prevention and treatment. Relaxation provided the antidote to the "enhanced responsiveness" of the nervous system, the sensitivity that is part of the migraine trait.

I first began practicing relaxation techniques myself—and the results were astonishing. Not only did my headaches decrease, but my sense of self-control, self-esteem, and general energy level improved. I also became aware that the source of health and restoration exists within each one of us. I wanted to extend this understanding to others and to use these techniques in my neurological practice. I saw this as a natural way to enhance medical treatment and improve well-being. I joined forces with nurse practitioner Donna Novak, a fellow migraine sufferer, and through our collaboration we found a way to integrate mind and body in the medical treatment of headache. This is the core of our practice at the Princeton Headache Clinic, and the essence of this book.

We invite you to join us to learn natural ways to prevent and treat headaches. If you can answer "yes" to any of the following questions, this book will help you find relief.

Do you experience recurring headache?
Do you wish to improve the effectiveness of your current medical treatment?
Do you want to use less medication?
Do you sense a loss of balance in your life?
Do you wish to have more control of your headache triggers?
Do you want to feel less stressed in your daily life?
Do you want to regain optimism?

This book is based on the success of the Princeton Headache Clinic *Headache Reduction Program* (HARP). HARP will teach you natural, drug-free ways to prevent headaches and to relieve the misery of recurring headache. These methods reduce stress, protect the nervous system, and restore harmony. They are timeless but scientifically principled techniques that can be adapted to everyday life.

As physician and nurse practitioner, our mission is to lessen the burden of the headache sufferer. As fellow migraine sufferers, we also have a personal interest in this work. Many of the patients that come to our clinic with headaches have also suffered from being misunderstood, misdiagnosed, and mistreated. Headaches are often not taken seriously once underlying pathology has been ruled out. The public and the medical community fail to recognize that although chronic headaches are not life-threatening, they are disruptive and disabling. Data published by the World Health Organization lists migraine in the top rung of diseases that severely impact quality of life. Clearly, people need more than an effective painkiller to gain control of recurrent headaches.

Our experience has shown that the people who gain the greatest control of their headaches understand what they can—and cannot—do about them. They learn to accept the part that is *not* in their control—that migraine is a biologic disorder of the brain and nervous system that predisposes them to having headaches. They have also accepted responsibility for the part of migraine treatment that *is* in their control. They keep a headache diary to track their headache triggers (such as foods, missed meals, and irregular sleep), and make whatever lifestyle changes are necessary. They stay in tune with their stress response and to the signals of an impending headache, and take steps to prevent the headache with techniques such as focused breathing, muscle relaxation, and positive self-talk. They also protect their nervous system and become more resilient to headaches with regular periods of relaxation, using such techniques as meditation, yoga, and mindfulness. They see health-care practitioners as partners in helping them achieve optimum health and well-being.

Part I of *Breaking the Headache Cycle* contains information about migraines, the nervous system, and stress. Part II teaches specific relaxation techniques and stress management strategies that will help you gain control of your headaches and live a healthier, happier life.

Origin of the HARP

Hi Donna!
I have not seen you in a while, but I just wanted to let you
know how I am doing. For the first time in about three
years I can actually say that my head does not hurt. My
daily headaches are virtually gone. Now I only get the
occasional full-blown migraine. Usually about once or
twice a month I have to stay in bed all day, but I can deal
with this much better. I am able to do normal things now!
I can do homework without pain and I even have extra
time to have fun and relax. It's great—I can make plans
now without worrying about how I will feel later on. I
never imagined I could feel this great!

I want to thank you and Dr. Livingstone for your help
and attention. I don't think I can possibly express what a
difference you have made in my life.

Sincerely,
Betty

Betty, age twenty, suffered from migraines and daily headaches
for several years. She recently sent us this e-mail from college, a
few months after completing our headache reduction program.

Edward, a fifty-four-year-old business executive, entered the program out of frustration. "I may as well try this—I have tried everything else," he said. He experienced severe headaches several times a week. Although he was able to control each headache with medication, he felt that he had no way to prevent them and sensed that he was always on the verge of the next one. He began practicing a relaxation exercise each morning before leaving for work. Within two months his need for medication dropped from several times a week to about twice a month—a dramatic improvement.

Evelyn, a thirty-five-year-old schoolteacher, found that her frequent headaches made her irritable and short-tempered with the children at school. She came to understand that this was part of her migraine trait that gave her nervous system the quality of "enhanced responsiveness." She successfully found a way to use simple breathing exercises. As she became aware of rising tension in her neck and shoulders, Evelyn responded by shifting the movement of her breathing to the abdomen (which reduces the tension held in the chest) and breathing rhythmically to a 1 . . . 2 . . . 3 . . . 4 count (this harmonizes the nervous system with natural body rhythm). In only a few minutes, Evelyn could restore her level of calm and prevent the rise of tension that may have culminated in a headache.

Betty and others benefited from four unique elements in our program:

1. Education and understanding of migraine is the essential first step in regaining control.

2. The clinic encourages self-care by respecting the body's natural ability to heal and restore. Medications are often not enough. Natural relaxation methods improve the effectiveness of and reduce the need for medication.

3. The program addresses the heightened responsiveness of the nervous system that occurs in migraine sufferers.

4. The isolation of the headache sufferer is relieved by shared experience. You are not alone.

The Limits of Drug Treatment

The biological tendency to recurrent headache is not easily remedied. A new class of drugs, called triptans, has revolutionized the control of the migraine attack. For some migraine sufferers these drugs may be the only treatment needed—particularly for those whose migraines are not frequent. Preventive medications are also invaluable in reducing the migraine tendency. However, there are side effects to all medications and limits to their effectiveness. Studies have shown that relaxation techniques reduce headaches to approximately the same degree as preventive medications. Relaxation techniques also enhance the effectiveness of medication taken for relief of an existing headache.

Natural relaxation techniques and medications complement and enhance each other. Our program uses whatever tools are necessary and safe to improve the migraine sufferers' quality of life.

The Role of the Nervous System

Many headache and migraine sufferers have a heightened responsiveness or reactivity of their nervous system. The sensitivity is part of the disorder of chronic and recurring headache. This trait is a double-edged sword, as it confers sensitivity to the good things of life but makes us more vulnerable to the damaging effects of stress. We are only now beginning to appreciate how much this hyperresponsiveness contributes to the misery and discomfort of headache. Medical treatment of recurrent headache is limited unless it addresses this heightened nervous system sensitivity. Relaxation techniques specifically tame this "enhanced responsiveness" of the nervous system and provide a vital aspect of treatment often ignored in medical practice.

You Are Not Alone

The people who enroll in the Princeton Headache Clinic's Headache Reduction Program (HARP) feel that there is something wrong, something out of balance in their lives. They come to the clinic for evaluation and treatment of headache, but most complain of being stressed out or burned out, of feeling driven and unable to relax. Some also suffer from frequent illnesses or chronic disorders such as fibromyalgia, irritable bowel disorder, high blood pressure, insomnia, or depression. They are seeking ways to improve their medical conditions without greater reliance on prescription medication. Many are taking medication and have tried other relaxation techniques such as transcendental meditation and biofeedback with limited benefit.

At the first HARP session, we ask participants to introduce themselves and talk about why they decided to embark on the program. Here are some of the thoughts people have shared:

"I want to regain some control. I feel I have lost control of my headaches."

"I feel guilty in having so many headaches. I feel I am failing others."

"Although the medications help me, I hate the side effects. Is there anything else I can do besides taking medication?"

"I feel stressed much of the time."

"These headaches are interfering with my life. I want to get rid of them."

"My preventive medications are making me gain weight. I want to find another way to control my headaches."

"I always feel on the verge of headache. There must be something wrong with me."

You have probably experienced similar feelings and thoughts about your headaches. As headache specialists and fellow migraineurs, we are here to say you are not alone and that there is hope.

Through the stories and words of our group participants, we will try to transmit some of the wonderfully supportive energy that a group experience generates and tell you how you may gain the same benefits as an individual.

2

Understanding Your Headaches

Barbara, forty-three years old, is a busy homemaker. She went to her doctor because she had experienced an increase in what she thought were her sinus headaches. Her ENT physician referred her to us after her sinus X rays were normal. Barbara's headaches, which she had been partially controlling with over-the-counter sinus medications, are now disabling. She can no longer function during a headache. She has to cancel appointments and find someone to help with her children's activities. She feels bad. She becomes more irritable and short-tempered during an episode. Her headaches, which now occur three or four times each month, begin over the right forehead and are made worse with movement such as bending forward; they make her feel nauseated. She becomes extremely sensitive to light and sound during the headache, which lasts up to forty-eight hours. Barbara has suffered with these headaches for twenty years, never obtaining relief. Her mother had a similar headache history at her age.

Jeffrey, age twenty-six, is a physics graduate student who sought medical attention after his third episode of visual disturbance and headache. These episodes begin with bright flashing lights in the right upper part of his vision over a period of twenty minutes, leading to partial loss of vision on the right side with wavy zigzag lines. The visual distortion is then followed by a pounding generalized headache lasting six hours, accompanied by nausea, light sensitivity, and inability to function. All three of these attacks had followed a stressful event such as a work presentation.

Claire, thirty-three, has been prone to headaches since childhood. Since starting her new job as a secretary for a very demanding boss, the frequency of her headaches has increased. They begin during the workday with a tightness and pressure that she describes as a "band around my head." If she doesn't take a painkiller her headache becomes more severe. She is now taking at least six aspirin a day to get by and has begun taking painkillers to try to prevent the next headache. Her headaches are less frequent on the weekends. She is seeking help for these headaches because the only advice she has been given is to "find a different job," which is not practical. She is beginning to feel like a failure for not being able to "cope."

These are three very different headache profiles that illustrate how difficult it is to understand and correctly diagnose the disorder that makes Barbara, Jeffrey, and Claire suffer. Let us see how these different headache types are related.

Understanding Migraine

Migraine and tension-type headaches represent the so-called primary headache disorders. There are other less common headaches in this category, including cluster headache and other rare headache types. We will not concentrate on these other headaches because they are well described in other books and are best treated with medication.

The tendency to have migraine headaches is lifelong and biologically determined. Many sufferers carry a sense of failure at not being able to "cope with life" and there remains the widespread misconception that migraines are all psychosomatic and that migraines are a mental rather than medical disorder.

Education about migraine is essential to successful treatment. Knowledge allows someone to be an informed decision maker rather than a passive recipient of care. It is the first step in gaining control. Understanding migraine also helps to focus on prevention rather than just reacting to each headache attack.

Barbara has migraine. When the biological basis for Barbara's headaches was explained to her, she broke down and cried. These were tears of relief and release from years of feeling that she was at fault and had failed to cope with life. Empowered with knowledge about her condition, she became an active participant in her care, making informed decisions about her treatment options. This was her first step to regaining control of her headaches.

Leave Your Diagnosis to the Experts

There are clinical criteria for the diagnosis of migraine and professional medical evaluation is required to make this diagnosis. Unfortunately, 59 percent of migraine sufferers do not receive a diagnosis until after seeing three or more physicians. This indicates that even education of physicians is still required. Despite this statistic, do not attempt to diagnose your own headaches. There are several headache types and medical conditions that may masquerade as migraine and it is essential that a medical diagnosis be made.

The Burden of Migraine

Migraine affects nearly one in every four U.S. households. Approximately 18 percent of women and 6 percent of men suffer with migraine. This translates to 28 million migraine sufferers in the United States.

Even though half of all adult migraine sufferers experienced their first migraine in childhood or adolescence, many remain undiagnosed. Based on a 1999 study, fewer than half the people with migraine headaches in the United States are medically diagnosed or treated. Many migraine sufferers are misdiagnosed as having sinus or tension headaches, and they rely on over-the-counter treatment. This ignorance also contributes to suffering. There is a sense of failure and guilt in not being able to "cope with life." This attitude results from the erroneous belief that migraines and headaches are caused by the inability to cope with the demands of life. This depiction of the neurotic headache is no better illustrated than by the comic-strip character, usually female, who feigns a headache as an excuse for avoiding intimacy.

This disorder affects individuals in their most productive years. The cost of missed work and reduced productivity from migraine is estimated to be $13 billion per year in America. Most migraine sufferers stay at work rather than leave, and they function with reduced efficiency. Migraine results in 112 million days of bed rest a year in the United States. Nearly half of the women and 38 percent of the men with migraine lose a week or more of work per year because of this disorder.

Definition of a Migraine

The International Headache Society defines at least six types of migraine as well as a category for "migrainous headaches" that do not fit into the main six categories.

The following are the criteria laid down by the International Headache Society and accepted by most researchers for migraine diagnosis. These are guidelines and are not a substitute for a medical diagnosis.

Migraine without Aura

Migraine without aura is defined as at least five attacks, each lasting four to seventy-two hours and consisting of at least two of the following characteristics of the pain:

1. Throbbing or pulsatile
2. Unilateral (one side of the head)
3. Of sufficient severity to impair function
4. Pain aggravated by routine physical activity.

Plus one of the following:

1. Upset stomach with nausea and/or vomiting
2. Increased sensitivity to light (photophobia) and/or sound (phonophobia).

Migraine with Aura

Migraine with aura is defined as at least three migraine headaches, as defined above, preceded by a specific disturbance of sensation.

The aura is usually a disturbance of visual function. This most commonly causes partial loss of vision, flashing lights (like "looking into a flashbulb," formed visual patterns, or moving waves). They may rarely be very complex. These visual disturbances have provided creative inspiration. For example, the visual distortions of Lewis Carroll's migraines are thought to have provided him with some of his ideas for *Alice in Wonderland*. Depending on which area of the brain is affected, the migraine aura may involve other disturbances of function such as numbness, loss of speech, or, in extreme cases, weakness. No aura should last more than sixty minutes, and the headache (as described above) follows the aura within sixty minutes.

Any neurological symptoms such as disturbance of vision, numbness, or change in speech requires medical evaluation and diagnosis. This type of migraine is more often correctly diagnosed because the symptoms usually prompt (correctly so) early medical consultation.

Jeffrey's headaches fit into this category. Jeffrey learned to heed the warning provided by his aura. He learned to let go and relax instead of tensing up in anticipation of his headache. By doing this and by taking appropriate medication, he was able to reduce the impact of the headache that followed. At times, he even prevented the headache from occurring. In chapter 7 you will learn ways to use the signals of a developing migraine to lessen the impact of the migraine attack.

The Stages of Migraine
Head pain is only part of the migraine process. A migraine attack may consist of several stages:

1. Prodrome
2. Aura
3. Headache phase
4. Postdrome

Dr. Edward Liveing, a nineteenth-century neurologist, described the types of migraine in wonderful clinical detail. He used the image of a storm as a metaphor for migraine: "The immediate antecedent of an attack is a condition of unstable equilibrium and gradually accumulating tension in the parts of the nervous system more immediately concerned, while the paroxysmal itself may be likened to a *storm*, by which this condition is dispersed and equilibrium for the time restored."

The thunderstorm analogy is appropriate. In fact, our choice of words reflects our closeness to nature. For example, we are "under the weather" when we don't feel well.

Let us see how migraines and thunderstorms are alike.

Early Warning: Prodrome

The migraine storm may be heralded by changes in mood, change in appetite such as carbohydrate craving, or by fatigue or yawning. These subtle changes may occur hours or even days before the attack. This phase, called the prodrome, results from shifts in certain brain chemicals that represent the gathering storm. We feel the storm in the air. We may feel it in our bodies. Often the gathering storm is confused with the trigger or cause of the headache. Barbara, for example, now understands that her sudden intense craving for sweets is part of her imminent migraine attack. Eating sweets is not a cause of her headaches, as she once believed, but her craving is part of the approaching headache storm.

The prodrome is the most subtle and overlooked part of the migraine attack. Not everyone will experience it. In chapter 7 you'll learn how to "tune in" to the subtle signals of the gathering storm and how to use this early warning to ward off the migraine attack. Intervention at this stage, with or without medication, can abort the migraine attack. You can learn how to use the subtle signals that nature gives you during the prodrome.

Lightning: Aura

As defined above, there are two types of migraine—with and without aura. In approximately 25 percent of migraine the headache is preceded by an aura—a visual disturbance of flashing lights or partial visual loss and occasionally numbness and tingling. This type of migraine is categorized as migraine with aura or classical migraine because the description dates back to antiquity—even preceding Hippocrates (400 B.C.). The most common type of migraine, not surprisingly, is called common migraine or migraine without aura. This is the old-fashioned "sick headache" presenting as recurring severe or disabling headache.

The symptoms of migraine with aura or classical migraine are usually those of the visual disturbance of flashing lights or partial visual loss and occasionally numbness and tingling. These sensory phenomena may be frightening at first. They may be dramatic and complex with complicated visual patterns and zigzag lines, or they may be simple with a "hole" or partial loss of vision called a scotoma.

Some people always get an aura before the headache. For most, it is a variable component of the migraine, occurring some of the time or not at all. Rarely, the aura occurs without any headache, in which case it is referred to as a migraine equivalent or ocular migraine. Many migraine sufferers, such as Jeffrey, can use the warning of the aura to avoid the sickness and pain that often follows. In much the same way, we run for cover when we see the lightning of an approaching thunderstorm.

The Storm: Headache Pain and Sickness

PAIN

The pain and sickness of the migraine storm arrive together. The pain varies in quality, intensity, and location. Usually it begins gradually, reaching peak within several hours. At times the pain is all over the head, but it may be localized to one side or in the forehead, where it is frequently misdiagnosed as a sinus headache.

Like the rolling storm with squalls of rain, the pain comes in waves. It is usually throbbing, synchronized with the pulse, but it may be pressing, piercing, or stabbing.

SICKNESS

Migraine is also known as sick headache. In addition to the head pain, much of the disability is caused by the accompanying sickness. During a migraine there's a loss of appetite, often with nausea and occasionally with vomiting. The part of the brain that normally filters out sensation malfunctions during a migraine attack. This allows sensations that normally don't bother us to become annoying. Smells, sounds, and light become highly irritating. Even the skin becomes hypersensitive. You may feel raw, exposed, and vulnerable during an attack. Your defenses are down, and you become immobilized. Peter, a thirty-year-old migraine sufferer, described the waves of his migraine attack like seasickness that he had once experienced. "At first I was afraid I was going to die. Then I was afraid I wasn't."

The Calm after the Storm: Postdrome
As the migraine subsides the postdrome, or aftermath, of the storm follows. It is usually experienced as feeling exhausted with low-grade head tenderness. Rarely, this postdrome is experienced as euphoria or a high resulting from the brain's production of intrinsic analgesics (endorphins).

These four phases of a full migraine attack are not always experienced during each migraine attack, nor are they experienced by every migraine sufferer. For some, the pain and sickness predominates, whereas for a few, the prodrome and aura are the main components of their migraine storm.

The Spectrum of Migraine
Some researchers feel that the migraine tendency is expressed as an array or spectrum of headache, and migraine sufferers often have more than one type of headache. On the one side of this spectrum, the headaches are mild and not disabling and may be called tension headaches. In the middle, the headaches are more severe, with features of both tension and migraine. This is often where the diagnosis of migraine gets confusing. At the other end of the spectrum the headaches are severe and disabling and are more readily identified as migraine. The tendency to different types of headache arises from the biological predisposition to headache.

Tension Headache

Because tension headache is not as severe as migraine, people with tension headaches seldom seek medical treatment. Simple over-the-counter remedies are usually effective. Headache specialists such as neurologists seldom see tension headache in practice unless accompanied by other more severe headache types or symptoms.

There are two types of tension headaches, the episodic tension headache and the chronic tension headache. These are defined by the International Headache Society as follows.

EPISODIC TENSION HEADACHE

Episodic tension headache is defined as at least five attacks where the headache lasts for four hours' to seven days' duration with the following characteristics of the pain:

1. Gripping or pressing
2. Not sufficiently severe enough to interfere with function
3. Bilateral (both sides of the head)
4. Not aggravated by physical activity
5. Not associated with nausea/vomiting or light/sound sensitivity

CHRONIC TENSION HEADACHE

A chronic tension headache occurs at least fifteen days of each month. Claire's tension headaches had become chronic. The stress of Claire's job increased her headaches but her underlying tendency to recurrent headache was biologically determined.

These definitions were drawn for research purposes. In practice, however, many headaches do not strictly fit into either definition of tension or migraine. For example, there are many tension headaches that are severe enough to interfere with function while some migraines are not disabling. There are now subcategories, which are called tension headache with migraine features, to better describe these headaches.

To make matters more complicated, most migraine sufferers have more than one type of headache. Tension headaches are more commonly experienced in people who have migraine as well. So the attempt to place different types of headache into neat little boxes is not always satisfactory. In order to explain this better, we need to understand the biological basis of migraine. The next section is a brief outline of our present concept of migraine-based headache.

The Biological Basis of Migraine

We now regard migraine as a chronic disorder of the nervous system. The intermittent expression of this disorder is headache. In other words, the headache is only part of the manifestation of the underlying biological hypersensitivity of the nervous system.

What Is the Cause?

The predisposition to migraine is largely inherited. Approximately 80 percent of migraine sufferers have at least one affected first-degree relative (parent, sibling, or child). The genetics of the migraine disorder are gradually being unraveled, and we are much closer to understanding the chemical basis of migraine. It seems that there are several genes involved—there is no one gene that explains migraine—a situation termed polygenic.

Based on what we know about the few migraine genes thus far isolated, the genes for migraine make certain synapses unstable. A synapse is a connection between nerve cells or the processes of nerve cells. At these junctions, or synapses, nerve cells communicate with one another by transmission of chemical neurotransmitters.

Certain groups of nerve cells in the brain become chemically

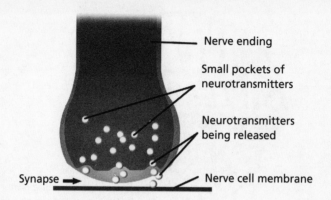

Nerve ending

Small pockets of
neurotransmitters

Neurotransmitters
being released

Synapse ➡

Nerve cell membrane

Figure 2.1   **The Release of Neurotransmitters across a Synapse**

unstable. These nerve cells, involved in the pain control system of the brain, have difficulty controlling certain neurochemical levels. The nerve chemicals, which act as messengers between nerve cells, are called neurotransmitters. They include serotonin and norepinephrine.

This instability of certain nerve cells is the biological basis for the tendency to have recurring headache. It is also the biological basis for the greater sensitivity of the nervous system in migraine sufferers. This is also the reason why many other medical conditions such as sleep disturbance, irritable bowel syndrome, premenstrual syndrome, anxiety disorders, and depression are more common in migraine sufferers. This will be discussed in detail in chapter 3.

When the nervous system becomes stressed or overloaded the neurotransmitter levels fall in the area of the brain containing these unstable nerve cells. This region can be thought of as the migraine generator. Discharge of these nerve cells activates a nerve called the trigeminal nerve, which carries sensation from the front of the head and face. This nerve terminates on the walls of blood vessels on the side and base of the brain and in the scalp. Once the nerve

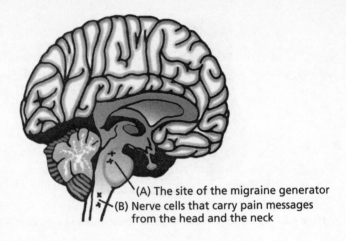

(A) The site of the migraine generator
(B) Nerve cells that carry pain messages
from the head and the neck

Figure 2.2   **The Migraine Generator**

The sites of unstable nerve cells in the brain stem. When activated, these cells stimulate nerve endings to release chemicals that dilate and inflame surrounding blood vessels.

is activated, chemicals are released from the nerve endings into the blood vessel causing inflammation, swelling, dilation of the blood vessel, and pain. This accounts for the throbbing pain of the migraine. The dilation of the blood vessel is part of the migraine process. It is not the initiating event, as was once thought.

In addition, the muscles of the scalp and neck become tight and contracted in response to the pain. This further feeds into the pain, preventing relaxation and reducing pain threshold.

Headache Threshold
Your resistance to getting a headache varies from time to time. How easily a headache is triggered is determined by this resistance, which is termed the headache threshold. Many factors, such

as stress, hormonal changes, and levels of nerve chemicals, set this threshold at high or low.

Once the individual threshold is lowered, a minor stress or trigger may induce the headache, whereas, at other times when the threshold is much higher, the same stimulus fails to result in a migraine. This variability accounts for some confusion and frustration in identifying specific migraine triggers. There is a difference between the cause of migraine (the biological trait) and the trigger (the occurrence that activates a particular headache attack).

For example, Marsha, a forty-year-old mother of two, suffers from common migraine. She is confused about her migraine triggers. On several occasions she has experienced severe headache shortly after consuming chocolate, while at other times she has eaten chocolate without any untoward consequence. She asks, "Does this mean I can never eat chocolate again?" The answer lies in this shifting threshold. At times (perhaps when she is more fatigued, premenstrual, or sleep deprived) she is more vulnerable to headache, and consumption of chocolate will then be the "last straw." At other times, when she is more resilient and her threshold is higher, she can probably do what she wants without much risk of triggering a migraine attack.

When neurotransmitter levels are stable, you are farther away from a migraine. You are then more resilient to headache—you are headache hardy. When the nerve cells become more easily activated as a result of unstable neurotransmitter levels, your threshold for getting a migraine is low—you are migraine vulnerable, and it takes less of a stress or trigger to activate a migraine attack.

You can see, based on this model, the distinction between the migraine trigger, which brings on any particular migraine attack, and the cause, which is the underlying neurochemical instability.

What Stops a Migraine Naturally?

Our own nervous system stops a migraine by quieting down the excited, unstable nerve cells and by bringing them back to normal. This inhibition of this nerve cell overactivity can be thought of as an off switch. This occurs naturally as the migraine runs its course. It happens most readily during sleep, which is why migraine headache is often relieved by sleep.

Migraine Is a Changing Disorder

In some people (we don't yet understand why) migraine gets worse over their lifetime. The headaches may become more frequent; the interval between the migraine headaches becomes filled with less severe tension-type headaches. This pattern is called transformed migraine, as the headaches transform from occasional to everyday. At the chemical level, there is difficulty engaging the off switch. Increasing use of painkillers aggravates the situation. When this happens, the headache can no longer be switched off and the sufferer becomes dependent on the painkiller. This state is called analgesic rebound and the headache comes back when the painkiller wears off.

Frequent painkillers provide confusing chemical signals to the brain, telling it that it does not need to engage the off switch. The mechanism for stopping the head pain now depends entirely on the painkiller. Preventive treatments usually fail unless the painkillers are withdrawn.

This transformational progression of migraine is an additional source of misery unless it is recognized and treated.

Treatment

The aim of treatment is both to prevent migraine and to relieve the symptoms when the attack occurs. Understanding migraine helps to appreciate how the different treatments do this.

The following is a summary of treatment options and how

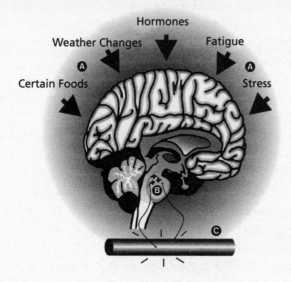

Figure 2.3   The Three Sites of Migraine Treatment

(A) Reduce or prevent the trigger
(B) Calm the unstable nerve cell
(C) Reduce the inflammation of the blood vessels

they work. Your treatment should be determined in partnership with your doctor.

Drug Treatment
Acute Attack

Anticipation of your next severe headache is a real source of disability. Living in fear of the next attack, you may find yourself withdrawing from social activity and commitments in case a headache strikes. You may do so to avoid disappointing others. Using painkillers in anticipation of the next headache is another avoidance strategy. It is natural to want to avoid pain!

Claire was doing this by taking painkillers before going out as her way of trying to avoid a headache. The strategy backfired, making her headaches worse and producing a condition of analgesic rebound. Getting control of the next headache is essential to any treatment plan.

This is an outline of how and where the treatments work. Details of drug treatments can be found in the reference section of this book.

The drugs used to relieve migraine are divided into four general categories:

- Anti-inflammatory drugs such as aspirin and nonsteroidal anti-inflammatory drugs (ibuprofen, naproxen, and many others) reduce the inflammation at the blood vessel wall and dampen the pain by doing so.
- Painkillers, such as acetaminophen and codeine, act by suppressing pain whatever the origin and are not specific for migraine.
- Ergot drugs such as ergotamine tartrate (Cafergot, Ergostat, Wigraine) act by attaching to receptors on the nerve terminal, reducing the release of inflammatory-causing chemicals and constricting the blood vessels. They have many side effects, such as nausea, and can aggravate vascular disease.
- Triptans are the first specific migraine "designer drugs." Triptans lock on to a receptor on the nerve endings, preventing the release of the inflammatory-causing chemicals and thereby relieving the migraine pain. These drugs have revolutionized the treatment of the migraine attack and often form the cornerstone of a treatment plan. The triptans are highly effective medications and, when used correctly under medical supervision, have a low incidence of side effects. These medications include Imitrex (sumatriptan), Maxalt (rizatriptan), Zomig (zomitriptan), Amerge (naratriptan), and Axert (almotriptan).

These medications are often effective in containing a migraine attack but, unfortunately, they do not prevent the next one.

Prevention

The preventive drugs act by inhibiting or stabilizing the unstable nerve cells that generate the next headache. There are many categories of these drugs, including beta-blockers, tricyclic antidepressants, certain anticonvulsants, and calcium channel blockers. Most of these drugs were found by chance to be effective in reducing migraine headaches, and all have potential side effects. Overall, research and development of the preventive drugs has lagged behind that of the drugs used to treat the acute attacks, such as the triptans.

Despite these facts, preventive medications are necessary and helpful in reducing the number of headaches in those migraine sufferers who experience frequent or uncontrolled headaches.

There is a downside, though, to taking daily preventive medications, namely, side effects. Often the primary effect for which the drug was developed now becomes the side effect. For example, beta-blockers were originally designed to slow the heart rate and lower blood pressure. Their use may cause sluggishness and low blood pressure when used to prevent migraine headaches in people who have normal or low blood pressure. Some of these medications also dull the nervous system. The increased sensitivity of the nervous system, which is part and parcel of the migraine trait, makes many migraine sufferers more prone to the side effects of medication. Our focus in this book is to explore natural ways that reduce the need for preventive medications.

Nondrug Treatment

You can harness the power of the nervous system to prevent and restore the loss of balance that occurs with a migraine attack by using your inner strength. This approach provides both an alternative to medication and a way to enhance its effect. These techniques can be used to both ward off a migraine and treat the attack when it occurs.

Acute Attack

Relaxation techniques enhance the effectiveness of medications taken to control a headache. The nondrug aspect should be part of the prescription. These techniques can ward off a developing headache as we heed the signals of the approaching storm, as described in chapter 7.

Prevention

There are two aspects to preventing migraine.

- Raising the migraine threshold
- Avoiding migraine triggers

The first is to find a way to raise the threshold for migraine, to make it more difficult to get a migraine no matter what the activating circumstance or trigger. The second is to identify and avoid, as much as possible, those factors that activate or bring on a migraine. The tendency to recurring headache, as we have seen, is biologically determined and, once aroused from its dormant state, is lifelong.

We can learn to prevent, in our involuntary or sympathetic nervous system, the accumulating tension and charge that lower our threshold for migraine and make us more migraine-vulnerable. This is how relaxation techniques can prevent migraine. Chapters 4 and 5 describe the role of the involuntary nervous system in stress and in migraine.

The other strategy to prevent headache involves awareness and avoidance of migraine triggers, as outlined in chapter 8. Elimination of some of the identified and controllable triggers may prevent a headache. Certain dietary factors, alcohol, skipping meals, sleeping too late, or not getting sufficient sleep can be controlled. In reality, there are many different migraine triggers; control over those that are easily identified may reduce the number of headaches but does not abolish the migraine tendency.

Claire obtained relief by stopping her aspirin intake and by using one of the preventive medications in low dose (in this case, amitriptyline) and learning stress reduction techniques that allowed her to adapt to her work stress in a healthier way.

Although natural methods give us ways to control and prevent headache without drugs, some migraine sufferers, like Claire, have such a degree of neurochemical instability that medications are needed for prevention. Ideally, once control is established and the headaches are reduced to a manageable frequency, attempts are made to substitute daily preventive medication with natural or drug-free ways to maintain balance.

Barbara and Jeff decided not to use preventive medications and worked with lifestyle and stress reduction techniques. Jeffrey, particularly, was successful at preventing most of his headaches as well as using his aura as a signal to relax. Both Barbara and Jeff became aware of natural ways to reduce their enhanced responsiveness to stress.

The Migraine Package
Many neurologists now view migraine as a chronic disorder of the nervous system, the intermittent expression of which is headache. The headache is only one aspect of the increased sensitivity of the nervous system in migraine. At the Princeton Headache Clinic, we call this underlying trait of increased sensitivity of the nervous system enhanced responsiveness.

This enhanced responsiveness accounts for why several medical conditions occur more commonly in migraine sufferers than in the general population. These disorders include insomnia, anxiety, stroke, irritable bowel syndrome, and premenstrual syndrome. The migraine trait is a "package deal" in that the tendency to headache is accompanied by this increased responsiveness of the nervous system.

Reducing the factors that stress or overload the brain can counter this heightened responsiveness of the nervous system. For example, migraine sufferers are very sensitive to changes in routine: shifting gears from high to low stress, skipping meals, hormonal changes, weather changes, and changing sleep patterns can all bring on a migraine attack. Studies have also shown that migraine-prone people have an exaggerated response to stress independent of the migraine attack.

This heightened responsiveness can be calmed and brought back to normal by using relaxation techniques. This makes the nervous system more resilient to stress and also helps to reduce the excitability of the nervous system that makes you migraine-vulnerable.

This answers the question "If migraine is a biological condition, why does stress reduction help?"

Six Points to Remember about Migraine

1. The migraine tendency is inherited. It must be managed throughout life.
2. Migraine is biologically based. It is not the result of poor stress management.
3. Migraine is still not widely appreciated as a significant medical condition.
4. The enhanced responsiveness of the nervous system, part of the migraine disorder, can be protected by natural techniques and lifestyle factors.

5. The enhanced sensitivity of the nervous system may manifest as one or more of several medical conditions that may coexist with migraine. These medical conditions can be improved if the migraines are adequately treated.

6. Migraines can be treated. There's a difference between treatment and cure.

3

The Gift: Enhanced Responsiveness of the Nervous System

Jennifer, a twenty-eight-year-old graphic designer, is frustrated by the frequent headaches she has had since she was fourteen years old. She gets a severe headache if she skips a meal, if she doesn't get enough sleep, if she sleeps longer than normal, if she travels across time zones, and if she gets excited—even for good things. "I cannot do anything off my routine without getting a headache!" she says.

Bill, a forty-two-year-old salesman, experiences severe headaches each Saturday morning. "I have a stressful workweek and I don't understand why my headaches strike when I relax on Saturday—it's not fair! "

Both Bill and Jennifer's nervous systems are very reactive to any change, even good change. This sensitivity is the hallmark of the migraine condition. Unless it is understood and recognized, the migraine disorder cannot be adequately treated. This lack of understanding also leads to self-doubt and erosion of confidence. "I feel there is something wrong with me—like not being able to cope with life," Jennifer exclaims.

That migraine sufferers are sensitive to change is reflected in the diverse migraine triggers that are a response to change. These include changes in routine, changes in stress level, and changes in the environment such as weather, light, sound, humidity, and internal bodily changes such as hormonal changes with the menstrual cycle.

Why This Enhanced Sensitivity?

The tendency to have recurrent headache results from a chemical instability in certain nerve cells in the brain stem, the lower part of the brain. We believe that the same chemical instability occurs in other parts of the nervous system. This enhanced responsiveness makes the whole nervous system more reactive and responsive than average. This trait contributes to the difficulties and misery of the migraine sufferer. In a more positive light, the same traits can be viewed as a gift. You can use this sensitivity to your advantage. You can learn how to protect your sensitivity and use this gift to enhance your vitality, joy, and health!

Why does a condition that causes such disabling headache occur in so many people? One of the theories as to why migraine has survived the evolutionary process of natural selection is that the enhanced responsiveness of the nervous system probably conferred some protection. Our early ancestors with migraine, particularly women and children, were more sensitive and alert to danger, slept more lightly, and were more responsive to environmental changes. This trait that may have helped survival long ago has now become a nuisance and a hindrance in a modern life where we are exposed to incessant demands, time pressure, noise, and all manner of constant stimulation.

How This Enhanced Responsiveness Manifests

Like our individuality, our sensitivity to change or stress is expressed in unique ways. It is reflected not only in the various headache triggers but also in the body. Let's look at some of the ways this enhanced responsiveness can manifest itself. These patterns, although uniquely expressed, are recognizable in clinical practice—I look for expressions of enhanced responsiveness in all my migraine patients.

Comorbidity

Comorbidity is a state in which several medical disorders coexist by association but where one does not cause the other. This comorbidity can be a source of confusion for patients and physicians.

Gina, a thirty-eight-year-old mother of two, has had migraines since her teens. She has seen many doctors for other complaints of abdominal cramps and diarrhea (diagnosed as irritable bowel syndrome) and for muscle pains and fatigue (diagnosed as fibromyalgia). She has three separate medical diagnoses and is taking several different medications. Gina felt like she was falling apart and that there was something wrong with her body. She enrolled in the group Headache Reduction Program and discovered that her fellow migraine sufferers also had other medical disorders. This understanding, coupled with the benefits of the relaxation techniques, has reestablished her confidence. Moreover, the benefits of the relaxation techniques and lifestyle changes have improved not only her migraines but also her other medical symptoms. She has been able to reduce her need for medications. Self-blame has been replaced by an acceptance of her biological condition that makes her vulnerable to these related but apparently separate conditions. Gina has learned to pace herself and to avoid being overloaded, and she has benefited from regular relaxation and exercise. She now views her enhanced responsiveness in a positive way—the same sensitivity that makes her vulnerable to these disorders is used to enhance her life.

In comorbidity, one disorder does not cause the other, but they tend to occur together. The disorders that occur most commonly in association with migraine include irritable bowel syndrome, premenstrual syndrome, anxiety, major depression, sleep disturbances, Raynaud's syndrome, mitral valve prolapse, social phobia, and bipolar illness. There is also an increased occurrence of epilepsy and stroke among migraine sufferers. The cause for this association is unclear, but the concept of enhanced responsiveness can go some way to explain this association. The increased reactivity of the entire nervous system (including the autonomic or involuntary nervous system, which is not localized to the brain but extends to all tissues including heart, intestinal tract, and vascular system) could account for the association of these different disorders.

Take depression, for example. There is an increased risk of major depression in someone who has migraine. The risk operates in the reverse direction as well. Someone who has a first episode of major depression carries a greater risk of subsequent migraine attacks. In other words, the depression does not result from having bad headaches, nor do the headaches result from being depressed. It is easy to make the mistake of using one condition to explain the other. For example, if someone is depressed and has migraine, it is a common error to say that the depression is causing the migraine. They may merely coexist in the same person. I have seen this over and over in my practice where the headaches persist despite successful treatment of the depression. Unless this relationship or association is appreciated, coexistence of psychiatric disorders with migraine remains a source of confusion to the physician and migraine sufferer alike.

The tendency in medicine and science is to think mechanistically—that one thing always causes the other. The limitations of this approach are evident with several unintended consequences.

- There is a loss of self-esteem and confidence because there is no appreciation of how the different disorders are related.
- The tendency to self-blame results because people feel

responsible for having so many things go wrong and for being so "sensitive."

- Treatment is directed to the isolated symptoms so that the "big picture" of the whole person is ignored in favor of suppressing or treating the various symptoms.
- When the underlying enhanced responsiveness is not addressed, the cycle of misunderstanding continues.

Sensitivity to Change

Many migraine sufferers know that change in routine puts them at risk for developing a headache. Sleeping later in the morning is enough to bring on a weekend headache. Not getting enough sleep can also do so. Skipping meals is a trigger for some, and this is often misinterpreted as hypoglycemia or low blood sugar. For many it is nothing more than the deviation from their routine. It has been said that the best lifestyle for a migraine sufferer is a dull and boring life! Of course we don't aim for this, but it illustrates this sensitivity to change.

Other changes that may trigger migraines include weather changes. Beth, who lives in New Jersey, often gets her migraines with weather changes. This relation to the weather in the past had been misinterpreted as sinus headaches. "I know what the weather is in Chicago," exclaims her husband. "When Beth starts with a migraine I know that there is a weather front moving eastward and that it is going to rain." Others describe themselves as human barometers. There is much conjecture as to how a change in the weather can trigger a migraine. For some it seems to be a drop in barometric pressure. For others, in different parts of the world, the ionic changes in the atmosphere resulting from a hot desert wind in the Middle East or Chinook winds in the Canadian prairie are thought to trigger migraine attacks.

Other changes that may trigger migraine are more internal. Hormonal changes in women commonly trigger migraine. The fall in estrogen levels that normally occurs premenstrually accounts for the frequent occurrence of migraine headaches in the premenstrual phase of the monthly cycle. Menopause is a time of life when many migraine sufferers see a change in their headache pattern, often with an increase in headache before a subsequent improvement.

Stress

Migraine sufferers are more vulnerable to sensory overload and stress. This does not always mean that stress triggers the headache but that the nervous system is more stress-responsive. A study performed by Hassinger and colleagues (1999) on college students shows this. A group of migraine sufferers was compared to a peer group that did not have a history of migraine. Each group was subjected to the stress of public speaking and to a second stress in which the hand was placed in a bucket of ice water for as long as tolerable. Responses measured included heart rate and blood pressure. The migraine group showed an exaggerated rise in blood pressure and heart rate in response to the stress compared to their nonmigraine peers.

Stress may be defined as the need to adapt to change. In this way the stress trigger for migraine may be viewed as another reflection of this sensitivity to change. The relationship of stress to migraine and nervous system is explored in detail in chapter 4.

Bill's history reflects a common pattern among migraine sufferers. The buildup of stress during the workweek is released in the form of his headache on the weekend. Bill's headaches responded to an adjustment in his sleep schedule—he sacrificed sleeping later and awoke earlier on Saturdays, mimicking the workweek, and practiced simple breathing techniques to reduce the buildup of stress while at work.

Many migraine sufferers are surprised that their headaches occur when they are relaxed. Bill's weekend headaches are typical in that his migraines occur in the letdown period following stress. I see the same pattern in the college student who successfully completes her term papers and the next day has a severe headache, or in a commuter, like Bill, who relaxes on the weekend, or a traveler who gets a headache on his or her first day of vacation. "It's just not fair" is a frequently echoed sentiment. Frustration of the letdown headache is also expressed by "Well, I'll just have to work seven days a week!" Fortunately, this does not have to be the case. How the change in pace of life causes a "letdown" headache will be explained in greater detail in chapter 4.

The occurrence of a headache following stress or once the challenge is met may have been one of the reasons that the migraine trait has survived evolutionary pressures. Our migraine-suffering ancestor, more aware and more sensitive to change and attuned to danger, was only immobilized after the threat had passed.

Becoming Easily Overloaded or Overstimulated

The sensitivity of migraine sufferers to sensory stimulation has been elegantly demonstrated in medical studies. In one study, an alternating checkerboard pattern of bright lights is placed before a migraine sufferer. The black and white squares flash alternately and, before long, the nerve cells in the part of the brain that responds to visual stimulus become increasingly active. This excitement spreads to more and more nerve cells until a migraine attack is triggered.

The same phenomenon can be seen outside the laboratory, when a headache is triggered by bright sunlight, by long hours in front of a computer monitor, or during a drive with flickering sunlight through the trees.

A similar sensitivity is seen with nonvisual stimuli. Strong odors such as solvents, perfumes, and cigarette smoke are known triggers for some migraineurs. This is not an allergy—allergy results from abnormal activity of the immune system. The migraine triggers reflect the sensitivity of the nervous system to certain forms of stimulation. This unique and individual sensitivity to stimulus is termed idiosyncratic. It is not quite understood how the nervous system becomes sensitized to certain foods, sounds, colors, or smells. We have come across some unique and unusual migraine triggers that can only be explained by this idiosyncrasy. For example, one person may get a headache triggered by the smell of pineapple, while another will by the texture of a certain fabric.

Sensory overload is the other side of the coin. Here, the stimulus is not unique or specific, but the quantity or degree of stimulation exceeds one's tolerance. When all the senses are stimulated beyond a threshold, one can become overloaded, often resulting in a migraine. Being in a crowd with bright lights and loud music is enough to trigger migraine in someone so predisposed. Migraine sufferers can also be overloaded by stress and demands. The effects of stress are cumulative. The enhanced responsiveness of the nervous system renders the migraine sufferer more sensitive to both the *quality* and *quantity* of sensory stimulation.

Emotion and Excitement

The triggering of migraine by intense emotion is often misinterpreted as a weakness or as not being able to handle feelings. This has led to the erroneous belief that migraine is a purely psychosomatic disorder caused by mental or emotional distress. This view has done much harm. It causes many migraine sufferers to hide their disorder, shield their sensitivity, and suffer in silence. It is one of the reasons that so many people do not seek medical help. No one wants to be told, "It is all in your head."

The sensitivity to emotion is part and parcel of the heightened responsiveness of the nervous system of the migraineur. This is reflected not only in how certain emotional states can trigger the headache but also by the more frequent occurrence among migraine sufferers of conditions such as anxiety disorders, sleep disturbance, and depression.

Some migraineurs protect their sensitivity to emotional stimulation by avoiding situations that would produce any emotional reaction or by finding ways to suppress their feelings. This is culturally accepted, but it may do harm in the long run. A pattern of avoidance often reduces effectiveness in dealing with life situations, and a chronic attitude of holding or suppressing feelings may lead to emotional dullness and even to health problems later in life.

The emotional part of the brain, called the limbic system, has close connections with the involuntary nervous system. This is why emotion is associated with changes in physical functioning such as heart rate, skin temperature, muscle tension, and breathing.

Excitement is often confused with emotion. Excitement is a state of increased energy or arousal and is more powerfully experienced when coupled with emotion. We can become excited without emotion when our senses are stimulated such as with bright lights or music played at a rapid tempo. The shifts or changes in level of excitement may trigger a migraine. The enhanced responsiveness of the nervous system makes the migraine sufferer more sensitive to the natural shifts in level of excitement and stimulation. Here again, many migraine sufferers find themselves avoiding situations—even pleasurable situations—in order to avoid the excitement and migraine that may follow. Fortunately, there are natural ways to harness this sensitivity so that life, with its ups and downs and exciting periods, can be experienced fully.

Muscles

Muscles—particularly those of the face, jaw, and neck—may also express enhanced responsiveness. Many migraine headaches begin with discomfort and tightness in the neck and shoulder muscles. Also, muscle tension headaches are much more common in people who have migraines.

Tightening of the muscles is one way we involuntarily defend our sensitivity. We use these muscles to hold in the emotions, to contain our excitement, to brace ourselves against pain. Clenching the jaw is common, as is grimacing. Some people hold their head and shoulders as if they're expecting a slap on the back of the head. For many the tension accumulates in muscles of the head and neck, and the tensing of the muscles becomes a habit; the ability to relax the muscles is lost. Phrases such as "carrying a load on my shoulders" or "a stiff upper lip" or "rock jaw" reflect ways of reacting to life.

Migraine sufferers may become afraid to relax these muscles for fear of what will happen. Some people seek relief from massage, which often works. However, a migraine may result if the massage is too vigorous, since the muscles have to relax gradually. The gentle stretching techniques combined with relaxation response as shown in chapter 7 can allow this to happen naturally.

Chemical Sensitivity

Certain chemicals have also been shown to trigger migraine by stimulating the senses. These chemicals can be found in perfumes, volatile oils, and cigarette smoke.

Chemical sensitivity is also seen in food as a trigger for migraine. Overall, these are less important than once believed. Current estimates suggest that approximately 8 to 25 percent of migraine sufferers have identified food triggers. Most foods that trigger migraine do so not by an allergy or immune mechanism, but by the migraine sufferer being uniquely sensitive to that particular agent. Some of the more common food triggers—tyramine, nitrates, chocolates, excessive caffeine, or caffeine withdrawal—act by dilating the blood vessels. Others do so by unknown mechanisms. Many migraine sufferers are disappointed to find that major dietary change does not always prevent their migraines. It is not fully understood why some people have significant food or dietary triggers and others do not.

One of the major problems in using daily medications to prevent migraine is that migraine sufferers are more sensitive than others to the side effects of drugs. Doctors who may not be familiar with this enhanced responsiveness in their migraine patients often cannot believe just how sensitive people are to medications. Very low doses of medication—sometimes ridiculously low— have to be used in some people. This sensitivity to medication is specifically addressed in chapter 6.

Advantages and Disadvantages of Enhanced Responsiveness

Advantages

In our modern fast-paced life it is sometimes hard to see what advantages there are to having a nervous system with greater-than-average sensitivity. This enhanced responsiveness of the nervous system may have conferred some advantage in the evolution of early man. Surprisingly, the headache itself may not have been an evolutionary disadvantage because it usually *follows* the danger, stress, or challenge. The migraine sufferer, modern and ancient, is immobilized only *after* the threat has passed.

This greater sensitivity or enhanced responsiveness not only makes you more reactive to external stimulation in your environment but also gives you greater sensitivity to your own bodily sensations and feelings. This sensitivity allows you to live with greater awareness and attunement. In Part II, we will explore ways to use this sensitivity to improve your quality of life.

This sensitivity can be put to good use with relaxation techniques coupled with awareness. It is from attunement or contact with the core of your being that you derive natural optimism, joy, and, even, love of life.

This core is your life, the sum total of your cellular and nervous system functions, soul, or essence. Whatever words we use, the feeling that results from awareness and contact with this inner or deeper part of yourself is what matters. The enhanced responsiveness of the nervous system, that which makes you more vulnerable to stress, stimulation, and emotion, is the same gift that allows you greater awareness and contact with your core!

Disadvantages

We live in a pressured society and are bombarded with sensory stimulation. We have to react to deadlines. Time pressures force us into unnatural sleep and eating patterns and leave us little time for exercise and physical regeneration in rest. Incessant noise and bright lights also bombard the sensitive nervous system. Under these conditions, this enhanced responsiveness can be a disadvantage.

The gift of enhanced responsiveness that once served us well when we lived closer to nature now becomes a burden. However, you can learn how to protect and nurture this gift without giving up the challenges and excitement of your life.

Headache sufferers often blame themselves for not handling stress well. Your sensitivity to change is often misinterpreted as a character flaw or inability to cope with life.

The frustration, and even sense of failure, is engendered by the attitude of society—including the medical profession—that tells you to "relax," and "get a life," or that medicates you to reduce your natural reactivity. These attitudes result from not acknowledging this enhanced responsiveness of the nervous system.

Ignorance of the enhanced responsiveness fosters self-blame and limits treatment to medications and unhelpful advice. When you see only the reactive or negative side of the enhanced responsiveness, you then place labels and make judgments that it is bad or harmful. This incomplete view ignores the whole package and just sees and judges the parts. This negative view ignores the life-positive aspect of your enhanced responsiveness—that which makes you more lively, aware, and sensitive.

If you do not know about this enhanced responsiveness you cannot understand why you are excessively sensitive to stimuli such as bright light, odors, and changes in the pace of life.

Of course, we are living beings with responsive nervous systems. The trait of enhanced responsiveness confers greater sensitivity to the nervous system. We like to think of this sensitivity in terms of the synonyms of kindliness, warmth, feeling, and sympathy. In this way it is an appreciation of and ability to respond to finer and softer feelings. Defined in neurophysiological terms, it is a lower threshold than normal for responding to a stimulus.

Your enhanced responsiveness is just this. The more sensitive your nervous system, the more you can react to your own inner impulses or to external changes.

What to Do about Enhanced Responsiveness

There are three general ways of dealing with the enhanced responsiveness.

1. Suppress the Symptom

When somebody has symptoms related to the enhanced responsiveness of the nervous system—symptoms that may include not only a headache, but also irritability, insomnia, anxiety, mood changes, difficulty adapting to changes in stress level or routine— the physician's tendency is to reach for the prescription pad. There are so many drugs that can suppress symptoms and so much economic and time pressure that make the "quick fix" so tempting. The hyperresponsiveness of the nervous system can be suppressed and dampened by medications such as antidepressants and tranquilizers.

No drug, however, is free of side effects. There is always a price to pay. That is not to say that the drugs aren't helpful and don't have a significant role to play in the management of symptoms.

Medications are an indispensable tool in preventing and relieving migraine. At the Headache Clinic, we are not averse to using medication, but we dislike the knee-jerk response of prescribing medication as the first and only option.

2. Suppress Vitality

If your sensitivity is misinterpreted as weakness and your reactivity considered undesirable, your next choice is to suppress your vitality. You can prevent both the highs and the lows of living—the same highs and lows that can trigger a migraine and to which we react vigorously. This leads to a dull, colorless life. In trying to suppress this responsiveness, you are in danger of dampening down or depressing your life expression.

Life is expression and movement. When you habitually contain your movement and limit your expansion, you deny yourself your birthright to full and complete living. If you do this long enough, eventually there is the danger of depression or of giving up when you no longer feel the stirring and pulsation of our own life.

This is not a theoretical or abstract concept. It is very real! We believe that this may be the basis for the comorbidity of depression in some migraine sufferers. It is also, as we will see in chapter 5, one of the "traps" of excessive use of meditation and relaxation techniques where peace and calm is attained at the expense of our vitality.

However, there is a third choice.

3. Use This Gift of Enhanced Responsiveness

The same enhanced responsiveness that makes you more reactive to the world around you allows you to be more responsive to nature and to the natural rhythm of your own life. The guidance and instruction found in Part II will help you to find ways to remain pliant and supple rather than becoming increasingly stiff and lifeless.

The approach in our clinic is to integrate natural techniques with medical treatment. They are not mutually exclusive. In fact, they augment one another. We are always looking for ways to reduce the need for medications. Our first response and question to ourselves in planning treatment is always, "what is the best treatment for this person using the least medication?"

Migraine sufferers have a choice. You can see your enhanced responsiveness as a burden or as a gift of life. Your sensitivity can contribute to the misery of migraine or can be an asset to be valued, nurtured, and enjoyed. The choice is yours.

4

Stress and the Nervous System

Our office was eerily quiet after September 11. "We don't understand this." "What is going on?" These were the questions posed by our office staff following the horrible act of terrorism. We had expected a flood of telephone calls and needs for urgent appointments from migraine sufferers whose headaches had increased from the stress of September 11. This did not happen. Many of our patients with frequent and difficult-to-control migraines experienced a temporary remission. It was only after two weeks that we noted a trend toward more severe and frequent headaches in our migraine patients.

Based on my understanding of stress and migraine, I should have predicted this pattern.

Headaches and Stress. Stress and Headaches

The words *stress* and *headache* are often mentioned in the same breath. What does stress do to the body? Why do many migraines improve during the time of greatest threat and worsen in the period following the stress? Why do some of us only get a headache during stressful times? Why do so many people believe that stress causes headaches?

The fact that a headache itself causes stress is often overlooked and misinterpreted. The fear and anticipation of the next headache is stressful. Trying to work or be productive during a headache is stressful. The pain of a headache is stressful. The increased sensitivity to light and noise is stressful. For some, the cycle of stress that follows a headache provides the stress that triggers the next headache—so a negative self-perpetuating cycle can be generated.

Only slightly more than half of migraines are triggered by stress or tension. Stress is only one factor that may unmask the biological tendency to have a migraine, but it is an important one.

To understand the relationship of stress and headache we need to know what stress is and how we respond to stress in both normal and maladaptive ways.

The Silent Epidemic

We use the word *stress* freely, without realizing what it is, how we react to it, and how damaging its effects can be. It is misused as a synonym for not being able to cope, for feeling overwhelmed, or for anything that just makes us feel uncomfortable. Stress, however, is a specific biological condition.

The relationship between stress and headache is easier to see than that between stress and other medical disorders. Because the nervous system in migraine sufferers is so reactive, there is often a short time interval between the trigger or stress and the onset of the headache. For other medical disorders, the link with stress is not so obvious—the accumulating burden of stress or stress load is a slow, gradual process that may take months or years to manifest in other physical disorders.

Like migraine, stress is a silent epidemic. According to testimony before the U.S. Senate subcommittee on Labor, Health and Human Services in 1998, 60 to 70 percent of all visits to primary-care physicians in the United States are for stress-related disorders.

The effect of stress on other "reactive" medical conditions is not limited to migraine. It can be seen in conditions such as asthma and arthritis, where the physical response to stress may result in a flare-up of the condition.

Many studies have shown how dangerous excessive and prolonged stress can be to our health. If stress is not reduced, it can not only increase your tendency to headaches, but also have an effect on cardiovascular function, the immune system, brain function, and the aging process.

There is evidence that migraine sufferers react more vigorously to stress than those without a history of migraine. This sensitivity to stress affects not only headaches but also the conditions that may accompany the headaches. For example, stress will exaggerate any coexisting anxiety or sleep disturbances.

This is why stress management techniques can help not just your headaches but improve your quality of life and health.

Headaches and stress are related in several ways.

- The headache in migraine sufferers often follows the period of stress. Bill's weekend headaches, described in chapter 3, are a good example.
- Headaches can occur during a stressful time. For example, during a tense meeting at work, a headache can develop. This is usually a muscle contraction or tension type of headache. Except for sudden and intense stress or emotional crisis, a migraine that occurs during stress usually develops gradually and begins as increasing muscle tightness and tension in the scalp, neck, and shoulders.
- Headaches can occur in anticipation of stress. For example, an increase in headaches may be experienced in the days or weeks leading up to a big event.
- Stress can accumulate and result in a changing headache pattern, usually with more frequent headaches. This may

account for some cases of "transforming" migraine in which the migraines gradually convert to daily headache.
- Stress leads to a change in perception of where we expect a poor outcome and where we become more negative. This changes our outlook on life and perpetuates the stress.
- The headache and the sickness of the migraine are stresses in themselves.

Understanding how you perceive and respond to stress gives you the capacity to select the best response to any stressful situation. You need to know how to use stress to your advantage and to combat it once it becomes your enemy.

What Is Stress?

Stress is a reaction to threat or danger. It results from the need to respond to the danger by activating your body to prepare you to engage (fight) or avoid (flee) the perceived danger.

We need stress to motivate us. This is so-called good stress or eustress. But, excessive stress (dis-stress) is harmful. The word *stress* is commonly used to describe both our reaction and that to which we react. Technically that which threatens us or forces us to meet a challenge is the stressor and the response that this elicits in us is stress. The stressor may be physical, such as exposure to cold or pain, or it may be psychosocial.

There are two scientifically studied models of stress that help us understand the real danger of accumulating stress: the stress response and learned helplessness. The first is what happens when we undergo stress in the short and long term. The second is what happens when we feel loss of control and helplessness.

The Stress Response

The biological basis of stress was first systematically studied by Hans Selye and brought to world attention in his first paper, published in 1936.

Selye, a physiologist working in Montreal, studied animals, mostly rats, in a variety of stressful situations, including exposure to toxic chemicals, exposure to temperature extremes, and other physical extremes such as making the rats run in a revolving treadmill to the point of exhaustion. He also studied the animals' response to mental and emotional stress, such as exposure to loud noise or extreme bright lights.

Based on these experiments, he described three stages of the stress response, which he called the General Adaptation syndrome.

- Stage One is the general alarm reaction when we are confronted with a critical situation. This is a call to arms and is the mobilizing of the body's defenses to meet the challenge.
- Stage Two is the stage of resistance, in which we try to adapt ourselves to the new situation. During this stage the body's defenses are maximized.
- The third and final stage is one of exhaustion, when we lose our resistance and succumb to the stress. This results in physical damage to tissue and, if the stress is not relieved at this time, eventual death.

Selye's genius was in observing that different kinds of noxious stimuli (heat, cold, chemical agents, psychological stress) would all result in the same three-stage physical response to stress, no matter what the stimulus. This finding was revolutionary in its time as it showed that the body has a predictable but limited response to stress.

Learned Helplessness

Curt Richter at Johns Hopkins University described an animal model for what he called hopelessness. Rats are very good swimmers, and they can swim for prolonged periods of time. In Richter's experiments, some rats were held until they stopped struggling or became immobile. They would then be placed in water. The rats that had been held drowned rapidly. It was as though they had given up; they were hopeless. Soon the language changed from *hopelessness* to *helplessness*. There are a variety of animal models for this. Basically, when an animal is subjected to uncontrollable and unpredictable noxious events, it learns that its behavior does not change the outcome and the animal gives up. These models are all about the loss of predictability and also the perceived loss of control resulting in a state of perpetual anticipation.

Stress and the Nervous System

The central nervous system is functionally divided into voluntary (conscious) and involuntary (autonomic) systems.

The involuntary nervous system controls our response to stress. It consists of the sympathetic and parasympathetic systems. In a healthy state these are in balance. These two parts of the involuntary nervous system are opposite in function. We need both for health.

The sympathetic system is the part of the autonomic nervous system that is activated in response to stress. Its activation leads to an outpouring from the adrenal glands of the hormones norepinephrine (noradrenaline), epinephrine (adrenaline), and cortisol (steroids), which results in an increase in heart rate, elevation of blood pressure, shunting of blood away from the skin to the muscles, and constriction of blood flow in the intestinal tract. It leads to a sensation of anticipation and anxiety. In 1941 Dr. Walter B. Cannon, a Harvard physiologist, coined the term *fight-or-flight response*. The fight-or-flight response is the automatic response triggered in the body once danger is perceived; it represents activation of the sympathetic nervous system.

When the parasympathetic nervous system is stimulated, on the other hand, there is a reduction in blood pressure and pulse rate, increase in blood flow and warming of the skin, and increase blood flow to the digestive tract. It is active when pleasure is experienced.

To differentiate between these two parts of the involuntary nervous system, remember that *s*ympathetic nervous system responds to *s*tress and the *p*arasympathetic is active when we feel *p*leasure.

Several factors determine how readily the sympathetic nervous system is activated. For example, evidence suggests that a low level of a major neurotransmitter in the brain—serotonin—enhances sympathetic nervous system activity and inhibits the parasympathetic. This may lead to an exaggerated rise in blood pressure in response to anger.

Stress reduction techniques are one of several ways to help reset this bias by lowering the tone of the sympathetic nervous system and raising the individual threshold for triggering the stress response.

The response to stress may be normal or abnormal/harmful.

The Normal Response to Stress

The normal response to stress has three stages:

1. Perception
2. Engagement of the autonomic nervous system
3. Results and effects of engagement

Perception

In the perception stage of the stress response, the stimulus is recognized as a threat. If the threat is known and recognized, then coping strategies are searched for. If it is an unknown threat, alarm bells ring.

Connections are developed in our nervous system that will engage the involuntary or autonomic nervous system. What

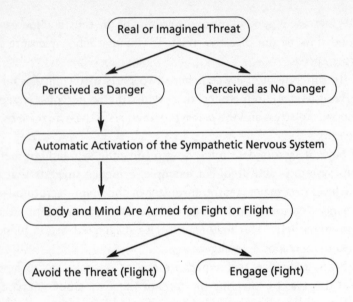

Figure 4.1   **The Normal Response to Stress**

may be threatening to one of us may not be threatening to the other—for example, a large dog approaching may seem menacing to me; whereas to another it is welcomed as an opportunity to pet.

Once we perceive a threat to our being, the emotional or limbic part of the nervous system is activated and this, in turn, engages the sympathetic nervous system in an involuntary response. As part of this reaction, our focus narrows on the immediate danger, and we become pessimistic, that is, we fear the worst. This has a protective effect (we do not talk ourselves out of danger—"that big tiger looks well fed and is not hungry.").

A superb example of how the mind and body work together is demonstrated by what happens when danger is perceived, even when danger is imaginary. This occurs in dreams or nightmares—

the sympathetic nervous system reacts with the same vigor as it would to real threat. We awaken from a nightmare with a cold sweat, a rapid heartbeat, and shallow breathing.

This response to perceived threat was hardwired into our nervous system early in our evolution, and it is seen in all animal species.

Fight or Flight

The fight-or-flight response is activated through connections with the emotional part of the brain and sympathetic system. This prepares us to meet the challenge with a flood of adrenaline and cortisol, increased heart rate, increased blood flow to the muscles, increased respirations, mobilization of the immune system, and a vigilant pessimistic outlook.

This response is an all-or-nothing one. There is no advantage to having half-measures in dealing with threat.

Effects

Once the stress is removed by our action of engagement or flight, we no longer need this heightened stimulation. The response is shut off when it is no longer needed and our state of readiness gradually returns to baseline. Our response to stress is protective and normal. We all need varying degrees of stress to keep us motivated and focused. Our growth and development come partly from learning to adapt to and meeting new challenges. We would not grow or strengthen if our life were purely stress-free.

The Abnormal Response

Our stress response may become damaging or harmful when it is triggered inappropriately (the hair-trigger response) or if we are unable to turn it off when it is no longer needed. Also, low-grade continuous stress leads to an accumulating stress load, which may eventually cause a breakdown in health.

Stress reduction techniques provide ways to manage each of these abnormal or maladaptive ways of responding to stress. We are dealing with a very primitive part of our nervous system that reacts in an all-or-nothing way. Once the danger is perceived, our involuntary reaction is the same. The same response can be triggered by many different stimuli. The abnormal response is one in which the reaction is out of proportion to the actual threat.

There are several ways in which the stress response may become problematic.

Hair-Trigger Response

The hair-trigger response is not appropriate for the stimulus—for example, social pressure is not actually threatening. Perception is often distorted and we often feel trapped or helpless when, indeed, there are many other options.

A hair-trigger response is activated with minimal stimulus. Examples of this are snappy or irritable behavior or, to a more extreme degree, road rage. This is where the stress response is immediate and out of proportion to the stimulus.

Excessive Response

Our response to stress is excessive when we become immobile, frozen, or ill.

The response is exaggerated or inappropriate for the stimulus. This excessive response is part and parcel of the panic attack, where the "storm" of sympathetic nervous system overactivity produces an overwhelming response far greater than that needed to react to the stimulus.

Our ancestor, a caveman, is walking across an open plain returning home after days of hunting. Suddenly a large-fanged tiger appears from behind a boulder with bared teeth and hissing snarl. A sudden knot appears in the caveman's stomach, his muscles tense, pulse becomes rapid, skin is sweating, and breathing is shallow. He prepares for the worst: being attacked and eaten. As the tiger approaches, he decides whether to engage the beast with the small club or to run. He drops his club and runs fast on bare feet over sharp rocks, scarcely touching the ground and not feeling the pain of the cuts. He scales an enormous tree with the ease of a monkey.

Your nervous system may give you the same signals when you engage in something that produces anxiety, such as public speaking. You may feel your heart pounding and skin sweating; you may look for a handy tree to climb. Obviously you are not in danger of being eaten, but your nervous system reacts with all the vigor as if you were. An extreme example of excessive or overwhelming response would be sudden death—people have been known to die of fright.

The psychological counterpart of excessive response is the tendency to catastrophize. Here, everyday stresses are blown way out of proportion.

Inability to Turn It Off

If the stress response is not shut off once the stress is over, the physiological changes persist long after the stress has passed. For example, some people have persisting raised blood pressure after the stress of a mental arithmetic test or public speaking. This is also seen when having the difficulty of letting go of issues and situations that continue to bother us long after their resolution.

Some Never Learn

Repeated exposure to small but identical stressors usually leads to a lessening of the stress response over time. This is called habituation. For example, once we get over the fear of public speaking and gain confidence, our bodies do not respond as if threatened. Some people are unable to develop this tolerance and never lose their stress response to repeated situations.

Repetitive stress, particularly with abnormal or maladaptive stress response, may lead to exhaustion, loss of energy, and the familiar burned-out syndrome. Anxiety, worry, and anticipation of stress primes the stress trigger; if ongoing, it adds to the cycle of stress.

Negative thinking is part of the stress response. If this becomes a habit, thinking becomes distorted. This cognitive distortion produces a feeling of anticipation, which lowers the threshold for the stress response—leading to a cycle of exaggerated responses.

Once the stress load accumulates beyond a certain tolerable level, malfunction in the body appears. The type of breakdown depends on the particular biophysical and genetic makeup of each person. The specific malfunction may manifest in the nervous system, immune system, wound healing, anxiety, insomnia, and migraines (in headache-prone individuals).

The Special Situation of Migraine and Stress

The abnormal types of stress response are not specific to any headache pattern, nor do they predict any particular headache pattern. Rather, the accumulating response to stress affects the migraine sufferer in unique and individual ways. Migraine sufferers have a particularly unusual response to stress in that the migraine episode often occurs in the letdown following stress. It is almost as though the stress accumulates in the nervous system and is discharged by neuronal and vascular overactivity in the letdown period.

The Misery of Chronic Migraine

The World Health Organization published a large study in 1997 called the Global Burden of Disease Study in which chronic migraine is ranked in the top four most disabling medical conditions—together with quadriplegia, active psychosis, and depression. The findings of the study took many by surprise. After all, migraine is not a life-threatening condition. Most migraine sufferers lead productive lives. Why does migraine cause so much misery? The relationship of the sensitive nervous system to stress explains a good part of this. Migraine sufferers often come to see their life through their migraines—always anticipating the next headache even while recovering from the last.

Factors That Reduce Quality of Life
There are several important factors that contribute to the erosion of joy and quality of life for the migraine sufferer.

Lack of Control and Unpredictability
Not knowing when the next headache will hit and having no reliable means of relief lead to heightened anticipation. This is stressful. The unpredictability and the lack of control are two major factors that contribute to stress and may immobilize you—at one extreme, unpredictability and lack of control are the tools of terrorism. If you recall that 52 percent of migraine sufferers are not medically diagnosed or treated and have no reliable treatment options available, you can begin to see the magnitude of the problem. The anticipation of the next severe headache results in increased activity of the sympathetic nervous system, and you may become more contracted into yourself and afraid to expand and interact. Recall how the migraine often comes on when you "let down" or relax after the stress. Anticipating this leads to accumulating stress. Lack of control and anticipation of the next headache can lead to a sense of failure as you begin to doubt your own ability and strength.

The Sensitive Nervous System
The nervous system in migraine is, as you have seen, more reactive and more sensitive to changes, including stress. The faster pace of modern living with pressure on your time and energy takes its toll as you respond to demands by adopting a chronic

fight-or-flight attitude. Because of your sensitivity, the sympathetic nervous system becomes chronically overactive unless you take specific measures to protect yourself.

Change in Perception

Part of the stress reaction is to fear the worst. This negative outlook is the automatic and protective way of thinking that occurs when you are under threat. This can become a habit. As long as you remain in this mode, you will think negatively. You may begin to see events, demands, and even other people in a negative light, always expecting the worst. You cannot counteract this with positive thinking alone. Unchecked, this negative perception leads to a self-fulfilling cycle of more stress and more headaches. Your outlook becomes gloomier and darker, and you lose the capacity to feel joy and expansiveness while you remain in this contracted state of being. Taken to an extreme, this is like living in a state of permanent emergency.

Annie, a twenty-eight-year-old woman with long-standing migraine, describes what it is like to always feel on the verge of a migraine. "I was afraid to breathe for fear it would bring on a headache." Her normal daily activities had become a threat to her health and every change in her routine a potential enemy. Annie has learned to respect her sensitivity to change. She understands that her sensitivity to change is a result of a biological disorder called migraine. By using relaxation techniques and modification of her lifestyle, she has broken the cycle of headache—stress—headache. By becoming aware of her limits and learning to say no to things that would have normally triggered a migraine, she has regained her confidence and is more outgoing.

Fear of Letting Go

Many people, upon entering our group program, express fear of losing control and are afraid to relax. We have come to respect this. At first it was difficult to understand: Why should they fear relaxing? Why should they fear a pleasurable state of being? On the surface it does not make sense.

You may become so used to a state of siege and contraction—your chronic stress mode—that you fear the opposite. Sometimes letting go can result in a headache. Relaxation is feared because your state of contraction or withdrawal is your defense against stress and external pressure. Unfortunately, this contracted state also blocks access to your internal feelings and softer and gentler impulses.

There are many ways we "hold." Muscle tension in the face, jaw, neck, and back is common. We hold our breath in partial inspiration because full and complete outbreath triggers the relaxation response. We also hold on to attitudes of compulsive work and self-doubt. Excessive thinking is also a result of being in the chronic stress mode. We have all experienced difficulty relaxing because "thoughts keep running through my head." These are some of the ways in which our response to stress becomes structuralized in our mental and physical attitudes.

The prevailing cultural attitude of compulsive work ethic, guilt, and frustration is seen in the response of migraine sufferers when they realize the nature or cause of letdown headaches: "I just have to work seven days a week" or "There's no point in relaxing—I'll just get a headache." Most migraine sufferers who say these things don't really believe them, but it reflects a fear of what happens when they let go and relax.

Accumulating Stress Load

Dr. Selye's experiments show us what happens to rats when they are overwhelmed by continued and unrelenting stress. They become depleted and exhausted, eventually leading to organ failure and death. Humans are not much different. We soak up and accumulate stress. Eventually this results in physical symptoms and physical disorders. How this is expressed is determined by your genetic and unique physical makeup. For some it is reflected in high blood pressure; in others, by flare-ups of arthritis. For the migraine sufferer, it is seen in the diminishing threshold for headaches, resulting in frequent, more easily triggered headaches.

Accumulating stress is one of the factors thought to promote the transformation of migraine from infrequent periodic headache to more frequent daily headache. This pattern, which used to be called transformed migraine, is now referred to as chronic migraine and represents progression or worsening of the migraine disorder over time.

The effect of accumulating stress is also seen in the aggravation of associated conditions that accompany the migraine trait, such as sleep disorder or body pains in fibromyalgia. Part of this depleted state is chemical, due to declining levels of neurotransmitters in the brain—levels that were already more unstable to begin with in the migraine sufferer.

Hopelessness

If not checked, this accumulating stress load may result not only in physical disorder but a growing feeling of "what's the use" or hopelessness. Consider an animal placed in a cage. Initially the animal is wild and fights against restraint and captivity. It is angry at the restrictions placed upon its natural expression and freedom of movement. Subsequently the animal becomes passive and resigned as its natural exuberance and expression are frustrated. Our physical, mental, and emotional contraction in response to chronic stress is the cage in which we may find ourselves.

Stress in Medicine: The Resistance of Medical Practitioners to Dealing with Stress

The role of stress in contributing to illness is largely ignored in medical practice, despite evidence that prolonged or exaggerated stress is harmful to the body. There are two main reasons that account for such resistance to dealing with stress.

Most physicians are not trained to recognize and deal with stress issues. We are trained (and rewarded) by treating legitimate or established disease. In fact, physician services may not be reimbursed unless a diagnosis code for a disease state is provided to the third-party payer. The focus on diagnosis and treatment of established disease sometimes comes at the expense of disease prevention. We often do not address the avoidable factors, such as stress and self-destructive behavior, that contribute to disease.

The attitude of dismissing complaints not attributed to "real" disease is no better illustrated than the experience of many headache sufferers whose symptoms have been dismissed because they were not life-threatening, as if the reassurance of having a normal brain scan should be sufficient to relieve the headache.

The second reason is that we physicians don't deal with our own stress. The rite of passage of internship and residency is to make us stress hardy, teaching us to "soak it up" and "stay the distance." This is like basic military training. So we emerge from this training with few stress skills and little attention to our own self-care. How, then, can we give to others what we do not practice ourselves?

As a result, the role of stress in illness becomes ignored, disregarded. This omits one arm of treatment and self-care. Good medicine is and will always remain a blend of art and science. It is best when we use the technology not only to "cure and treat" but also to promote and support the body's natural ability for healing and restoration.

Relaxation

The opposite of the stress response is the relaxation response. We have the tools to restore balance by using what nature has given us. We can learn to use opposite functions to maintain health. The next chapter further explains the opposite functions of the sympathetic and parasympathetic involuntary nervous system. From this we learn ways to calm the nervous system and reduce the effects of stress—ways that augment medical treatment and help restore optimism, peace of mind, and joy of living.

Those biologically predisposed to headache may have a headache brought on by several factors including stressful events. In this case, stress reduction techniques make excellent sense. These techniques will also help even when headaches are not activated by stress events. This is because the heightened responsiveness of the nervous system, part of the headache tendency, can be calmed naturally. This raises the threshold for headaches triggered by other challenges such as weather changes, hormonal fluxes, and changes in daily routine.

5

Restoring Balance in the Nervous System

Most problems contain all the elements for their own solution. Thomas Troward, an English judge at the turn of the century, was interested in natural laws, including the power of mind and belief. He used the analogy of how iron floats on water to illustrate how a problem can be solved by understanding the underlying principles. A bar of iron will obviously sink when placed in water. The same principle of weight and displacement will allow iron to float if it is shaped into a boat. In a similar way, distress and disorder that result from stress-induced loss of balance in our nervous system can be restored by the same principle that caused the imbalance in the first place. Balance in the nervous system is a concept of function, and not literally a physical balance. This chapter explores these natural principles of balance and restoration.

Balance and Health

Health is more than the absence of disease. It is the natural state of harmonious integration of our organ systems, including the voluntary and involuntary nervous system. It is a state of ease and dynamic balance. Disruption of this balance results in a feeling of unease. If this loss of balance continues, it may eventually lead to disease.

In health, there is a balance between the sympathetic and parasympathetic nervous systems. This underscores the functional relationship—the relationship between opposite functions that helps maintain balance and our equilibrium. This use of opposing forces to maintain balance is seen in all body systems.

The Steady State

Claude Bernard, often called the father of physiology, had studied to be a surgeon. He became curious as to how the body maintained a constant equilibrium and adjusted to change. In 1846 he investigated how the involuntary nervous system functions to maintain our bodies in a constant state. He recognized the role of the involuntary nervous system in maintaining body temperature. He saw how exposure to cold causes the blood vessels of the skin to constrict, thus reducing the dissipation of heat from the skin surface. In hot weather, the blood vessels dilate, increasing blood flow to the skin and allowing for cooling by loss of surface heat. These opposite functions—the alternate dilatation or constriction of the blood vessels of the skin—serve to maintain a constant internal temperature and, in turn, are regulated by activity of the involuntary nervous system.

Approximately fifty years later Dr. Walter Cannon at Harvard referred to Claude Bernard's concept of a stable internal environment by coining the term *homeostasis*. This word is derived from the Greek *homoios*, for similar, and *stasis*, for lack of movement or remaining static. Dr. Cannon had begun studying intestinal motility in animals when he observed that intestinal movement ceased when the animals became frightened. This observation led him to study the effect of stimulation of the sympathetic nervous system; based on this, he described the fight-or-flight response.

The concept of homeostasis is that health lies within a range of function—"normal" values for blood sugar, cholesterol, blood pressure, for example, are expressed as a range and not as a single fixed value. The concept of a steady state means that we function within this normal range of health, but not at a constant level. We breathe, pulsate, move, and express. We expand in pleasure or contract under threat.

Sometimes this steady state is confused with stillness. Life is never stagnant or still. Our desire for stillness and peace may lead us to search for a state of constancy. As we will see later in this chapter, one of the "traps" of excessive use of relaxation and meditation techniques is to strive for the ideal of complete quiet with stillness for prolonged periods of time.

Balance and the Autonomic Nervous System

The concept of balance by opposing functions has been represented by heaven-earth, positive-negative, and the ancient Chinese concept of yin-yang. This same principle exists as the two divisions of the autonomic nervous system, which has close connections with the limbic or emotional part of the brain.

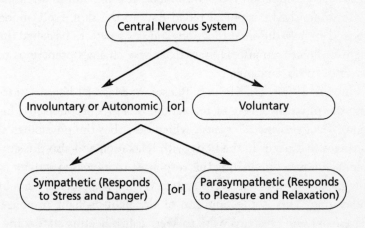

Figure 5.1   **The Nervous System**

The two divisions of the autonomic nervous system are the sympathetic and parasympathetic, which are anatomically and functionally distinct from each other.

The sympathetic nerves originate in the brain and emerge from the thoracic (middle) spine and lumbar (lower) spine. These nerves use norepinephrine as their chemical messenger or neurotransmitter. The parasympathetic nerves emerge from the brain and sacral (tail) spine and use acetylcholine as their neurotransmitter. Both the sympathetic and parasympathetic nerves accompany the spinal nerves and blood vessels branching into a smaller and finer network that enter and surround our internal organs, blood vessels, and skin. This autonomic nervous system is a vast network of fine, delicate fibers throughout the entire body. Activation of the sympathetic or parasympathetic nervous system has far-reaching effects.

Rather than risk becoming lost in details of each function, let's stand back and look at the larger perspective of how the nervous system works. Walter Cannon's experiments are helpful in this regard. Stimulation of the sympathetic system results in increased heart rate, respiration rate, and blood pressure, and in sweating with diminished peripheral blood flow to the skin. Dr. Cannon looked at these different functions and saw a pattern he called the fight-or-flight response. He saw that these changes prepare us to meet or run from danger.

In the 1960s, Dr. Herbert Benson at Harvard began studying the physical effects of relaxation. In 1975 he published his book *The Relaxation Response*, which describes the physiological changes that occur in the body with relaxation and also the simple techniques for eliciting this response. An increased activity of the parasympathetic nervous system is the physiological basis of relaxation. This is the opposite of the fight-or-flight response. These opposing systems work to keep us in a healthy state somewhere between stress and relaxation. We function in a narrow range between the two.

As much as we would like to be constant, still, and at peace, this is seldom possible. Moment to moment we move, we change, our perceptions change, and our bodies react. Even sleep is not a constant state, as we respond to dreams, move about, and toss and turn with microarousals through all stages of the sleep cycle. The movement within this normal range is maintained by opposite functions.

We can think of the two parts of the autonomic nervous system as the two ends of a pair of tweezers or the opposing movements of our thumb and index finger when we pick up a tiny object. These two opposing forces direct our function and energy in a particular direction and allow for precision of movement and give us a delicate touch. The same principle of fine opposing forces produces the steady hand of the surgeon or the artist.

We can also view this as a pair of scales—like an old chemical balance.

What Changes This Balance in the Autonomic Nervous System?
In health, the balance between the two opposite functions of the involuntary nervous system is not fixed and rigid. It swings depending on which component predominates at any one time.

FACTORS THAT INCREASE THE SYMPATHETIC
NERVOUS SYSTEM TONE
The activity of the sympathetic nervous system is increased with stress or when we meet challenge. Activation of the sympathetic nervous system brings us to a state of heightened readiness and mobilizes all our defenses. In this state, we are unable to rest or relax, and healing and restoration are put on hold.

We all have different normal and abnormal stress responses. The abnormal response may produce excessive or prolonged activation of the sympathetic nervous system. The way we deal with our inner impulses and emotions can also result in prolonged

Health Functioning
The sensitive balance—the load is light.

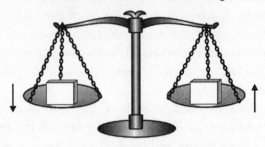

Chronic Stress and "Burnout"
The balance is less sensitive—the load is heavy.

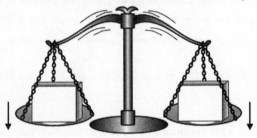

Figure 5.2   **Achieving Balance**

activation of the sympathetic nervous system. This is the physical basis of worry, anxiety, and restlessness.

FACTORS THAT INCREASE THE
PARASYMPATHETIC NERVOUS SYSTEM TONE
Sinking into your favorite comfortable chair at the end of a day's work, relaxing on a beach, falling asleep, eating a leisurely meal, and enjoying physical intimacy all involve activation of the parasympathetic nervous system. This is the relaxation or pleasure component of the autonomic nervous system. Like stress, it can be taken to an extreme, where excessive relaxation can reduce vitality.

How Sensitive is This Autonomic Nervous System Balance in Migraine?

The sensitivity of your internal balance is largely determined by the reactivity and sensitivity of the nervous system. Like an old chemical balance, fine changes result in a swing of the scales. The increased reactivity or enhanced responsiveness of the nervous system in migraine-prone individuals renders this balance more delicate and sensitive. Here, the sympathetic nervous system is more reactive and, if unchecked, will predominate. If this happens, balance is lost in favor of increasing sympathetic tone. We become chronically more reactive, resulting in a narrower range of normal function. It takes less change or stress to disturb well-being and take us out of this normal range.

For example, Joseph, a twelve-year-old boy with migraine, always gets a bad headache if he stays up late at night and does not get enough sleep. Even going to bed two hours later than normal will result in a headache. His sister Sarah, age fourteen, does not suffer with headaches and can stay up late with her friends without any undue consequences apart from feeling tired the next day. Joseph sees this difference. "It is not fair!" he exclaims angrily. Joseph's sensitive nervous system is more reactive to changes in his routine and places limits on his range of function.

Migraine sufferers require a greater level of vigilance to maintain the balance of their autonomic nervous systems.

Stress Resistance

The concept of balance can help you understand how to become more stress hardy. In short, your stress hardiness depends on how well you prevent overtipping of the balance.

You can make the balance more resistant to change by becoming less sensitive or you can respect your sensitivity and maintain balance by frequent small adjustments.

You can achieve balance in one of two ways:

- Make the balance less reactive, or
- Restore balance

Make the Balance Less Reactive

One way you can protect yourself when you feel overloaded or are stressed to the maximum is to "shut down." We do so to protect ourselves and make ourselves less sensitive. This is an emergency protective measure that can also result from prolonged and accumulating stress.

The sensitivity of the nervous system is reduced when you feel burned out or numb, and you can become less reactive, less feeling, and less sensitive.

Medication can dull or reduce the sensitivity of the nervous system.

Restore the Balance

You can make frequent minor adjustments to maintain balance before it is too late. This response requires awareness and perception. This is the basis of the attunement or awareness that comes with the practice of relaxation methods.

Make the Balance Less Reactive—
Reduce the Sensitivity of the Scales

Burnout

Burnout is a state of exhaustion or depletion that results from chronic and continued stress without relief.

Joy, forty-six years old, is a single parent who works full-time to support her three children. She has very little free time and skips sleep in order to get the housework done. Her migraines, which used to occur every few months, have become daily. She is taking analgesics every day to "keep going." She complains of feeling exhausted. She knew something was out of balance and was looking for a more enduring solution than antidepressant medication. Her headaches responded to low doses of preventive medication and reduction of her painkillers. Stress reduction techniques provided her the greatest relief. She learned, for example, that periods of relaxation and restoration improved her well-being. She learned that time set aside for self-care is not self-ish or self-indulgent but necessary for health. As she found ways to reduce the impact of stress on her body, she restored the sensitivity of her inner balance.

The reduction in your sensitivity as your burden and load increases is illustrated by what is known as Weber's Law. This helps us understand the different ways of maintaining balance.

Weber's Law states that our sensitivity to change is proportional to the level of stimulation. For example, if you are carrying a sack of potatoes, you will not feel the weight of a penny added to the load. If you are carrying a feather, the added weight of a penny will be immediately obvious.

When we carry a heavy load, or are chronically stressed, we hardly notice the addition of new stressors. The stress load we carry reduces our sensitivity to change and balance. The same principle is reflected in our body—when poor posture becomes a habit, we lose awareness of our slouching and bent shoulders. We lose our ability to make small fine adjustments that keep our spine aligned and in balance.

Most of us adjust and maintain balance at a completely unconscious level. We do so automatically. We have no way of changing our reaction to stress as long as we remain unaware of how we react. As a rule, increasing stress leads to diminishing awareness.

See how some people look as though they are carrying a heavy burden on their shoulders when stressed. They look "heavy." We often refer to stress in terms of physical weight and color. Compulsive work, no respite, and little joy leads to a heavy and colorless existence.

With diminishing sensitivity to our needs, our own bodies become more and more bowed until some aspect of our function gives out—such as backache or a slipped disk.

When we carry a heavy stress burden, we may not notice additional stress added to the load. We fail to avoid this additional stress and we neglect ourselves. Sometimes we begin to "sacrifice" ourselves for others, for a job, and so on. This reduction in sensitivity protects us in the short term as it allows us to get through a crisis or emergency. However, if it is unchecked, the stress load accumulates, leading to physical disorder or burnout.

In the burnt-out state we have become used to continuous activation. On several levels this results in depletion that is manifested as a lack of energy, joy, and vigor. The depletion of neurotransmitter chemicals in the nervous system—including serotonin and norepinephrine—leads to depression, anxiety, increased sensitivity to pain, and pessimism. At this stage, the stage of early exhaustion, many turn to medications for help. Most of the antidepressant drugs act to raise up the neurotransmitter levels in the brain.

These drugs are helpful but in some cases are used to merely blunt the signals of stress. In this way many people keep on functioning in the stress mode as the balance becomes less and less sensitive and the scales slowly tip. Without learning to take natural periods of rest and recovery, the state of exhaustion is masked and continues. We can learn how to prevent our nervous system · from becoming this depleted. The same principle (Weber's Law) that can cause us to feel heavy and burdened can also be used to lighten our load.

Drugs

In the era before modern pharmacology, the few available medications were nonspecific sedatives such as bromides. They were used to treat a variety of complaints from anxiety to psychosis to epilepsy. These drugs dulled the entire nervous system. The newer, more potent drugs are much more selective for specific chemicals or chemical receptor sites in the nervous system and are increasingly used in medical practice to treat the effects or symptoms of stress.

Chronic stress causes a loss of balance between the sympathetic and parasympathetic systems. In overdrive the sympathetic is dominant (sympatheticotonia). The restoration of the balance can be attempted pharmacologically by reducing the sympathetic overdrive.

Most medications that reduce or blunt the effect of stress do so by dampening the sympathetic tone. The effect is not limited to reducing the sympathetic nervous system activity. These medications also have some effect in reducing the responsiveness of the whole nervous system. No medication is 100 percent selective for only the abnormally increased sympathetic activity. The trade-off for reducing the tendency to the fight-or-flight response is often a dulling of the nervous system and a reduction in the sensitivity of the intrinsic balance. While this dulling effect is not as obvious as with general sedatives drugs, it does occur.

Restoring the Balance—Maintaining Our Sensitivity

Can you apply the principle of Weber's Law to keep the load light and balance sensitive? This is the more natural way of restoring and maintaining balance. We see three ways to do so.

- Listening to your body
- Taking periods of rest and relaxation
- Making changes, taking action

Learning to Listen

Again, by applying Weber's Law, you can maintain balance by making frequent small adjustments to keep the load light. You maintain your sensitivity to change by being aware and able to listen. This awareness consists of a process of inner listening or attunement. Whatever name we use to describe it, it is a process of feeling and perception. You can learn how to break out of the stress mode and regain a capacity for making contact with your own biological core or life center. You do so by learning to listen. This capacity for awareness is vital to your well-being.

One effect of repeated stress is that you focus on the external or perceived threat, always reacting. You thereby lose the feeling or awareness of what the body tells you. Stress reduces your capacity for feeling because it numbs you and makes your expectations negative. While in the stress mode, you focus on the external stress or danger, and no longer pay attention to the fine and sensitive signals from your own body. As you ignore these feelings you override your need for rest and reflection. Without feeling what is necessary for health, you may add to the cycle of stress by adopting poor health habits such as eating a high-fat diet and consuming toxins such as tobacco and alcohol.

There are several consequences to not being aware of your bodily feelings and sensations.

1. You have a diminished ability to feel the sensations by which the body tells you what is needed for recovery and healing.
2. You are less capable of acknowledging your need for rest, recovery, and regeneration. You neglect yourself, as you remain focused on external issues, circumstances, and perceived threat.
3. With accumulating stress, you lose the capacity to appreciate the signals of losing balance. The loss of balance in your nervous system is perceived as unease, a feeling of restlessness, or anxiety.
4. Continued neglect of yourself with lack of self-care and respect for the body eventually leads to disease.

By contrast, when you regain the ability to feel your bodily sensations:

1. You learn what is best for the body (it tells you).
2. Optimism is recovered because true optimism arises from deep within, from your own biological core.
3. You learn that your strength resides within—for the same reason.
4. Your resistance to stress increases as you become less rigid and more flexible.
5. Your sympathetic nervous system becomes quieter.
6. You place a greater value on your vitality and health.

Periods of Rest

Often we only take a break when we're depleted or exhausted, but it's important to remember that regular periods of rest and relaxation are restorative and necessary to help maintain our balance. They are not selfish or self-indulgent. Rest is a state of withdrawal from activity that engages the sympathetic nervous system thus allowing the parasympathetic nervous system to become more active. This may include withdrawal from physical activity, such as taking a nap, or being physically active in tasks that give pleasure, such as exercise, creative activities, or social interaction.

Relaxation is not only physical rest but also mental rest. You can take advantage of the relaxation mode by using and enjoying your awareness and the receptivity that results from the process. This awareness, or deep silent listening, further deepens the relaxation response. It is also called passive awareness—not a dulling and not a disregard of the body, but an immersion into your body wherein your intuition, guidance, and intelligence reside. This happens when you begin to listen, and you listen best when relaxed and receptive.

Periods of rest are important to recharge and regenerate the body and mind. Cycles of activity and rest are a part of life and nature. When stressed, you restore your balance through periods of relaxation. When injured, you need rest to recover. The healing of a simple sprain or cut provides an example. The stressed or injured part is rested, allowing natural intelligent function to restore and heal. This is a natural spontaneous activity, but if you do not give it a chance (keep walking on the sprained ankle!), the restoration does not happen as quickly or as well. The point here is that when you remove the obstacle to healing, the restoration of natural function occurs spontaneously. A research group at Ohio Sate University College of Medicine, led by Dr. Janice Kiecolt-Glaser, has demonstrated that simple skin wounds heal more slowly when we are stressed.

Most relaxation methods involve quieting your overactive mind and tuning in to your natural rhythm. As you will see in chapter 8, you can use your natural breathing to relax. Awareness of the breath is the link between mind and body. The breath provides one source of internal biofeedback, the feedback from our own cells! It is always with you wherever you go and provides you immediate access to your own internal rhythm and ability to restore and maintain your sensitive balance.

Decreasing External Stress, Taking Action, Making Changes
As you have seen, stress affects your perception and narrows your focus. Your stress load increases significantly when you feel trapped and when you see few options. It is greatest when you are unable to make meaningful changes to reduce the source of stress. The stress mode prevents you from seeing the big picture as you focus narrowly on the challenge or threat.

In contrast, when you are in the relaxed state, your perception broadens and you can see your options more clearly. This prevents you from feeling trapped and gets you out of the cycle of stress-induced negative thinking. You are then able to pick out the most efficient ways to respond to the stress. Instead of feeling like "it's no use" or "I can't do it," you respond to a stressful situation by thinking "Let me see what caused this problem in the first place" or "I'll ask for advice."

This does not mean that you have to give up the challenges of a demanding job or working toward an ideal or realizing your ambitions. All worthwhile achievement requires effort and work. Once you become aware of the options, you are always reviewing and evaluating your priorities. This awareness of options alone— being able to make choices—will reduce stress.

Robert Sapolsky, professor of biology at Stanford University, has studied baboon colonies in Kenya. His studies show how perception and social position in the animal kingdom influence the stress response. The baboons at the lowest rung of the social order, with the least coping skills and fewest options, show the greatest stress. The level of stress manifests with high levels of stress hormones and, like their human cousins, the development of accelerated coronary artery disease.

Stress reduction not only involves relaxation and awareness but the ability to make changes, to take action. By first freeing your mind from the stress reaction, you are then able to take useful and corrective action. This results in a positive cycle of relaxation, leading to greater awareness and then intelligent and constructive action.

In this way the changes you make to your life are constructive and life enhancing. They are not merely reactive. For example, one of the greatest stress factors in modern life is time pressure. Management of our precious free time becomes an important stress reduction tool. Cutting out unnecessary activities and using some time each day for self-care helps maintain our balance. Taking a walk on a summer evening after work to clear the mind and to listen is a healthier alternative than slumping in a chair and watching television. Changing evening habits, such as avoiding frantic work at bedtime or not staying up to watch television while exhausted, promotes more restful sleep. When you make these changes you will become aware of what you need to remain healthy and vigorous.

Another option is to limit your exposure to negative or

emotionally draining people where possible. Again, this is *not* selfish but necessary. You may have to give yourself "permission" to do these things.

Biofeedback and Lie Detectors

Most of us have forgotten what it feels like to relax! You may think you are relaxing, but you still have imbalance in the sympathetic and parasympathetic nervous system. With chronic stress we lose awareness of the subtle and fine body signals that indicate our level of stress and discomfort. We override the signals and sensations.

You may have lost your capacity to tune into these fine signals. Stress becomes a habit, a way of life. When you get to this stage, you may need some help to relearn what it feels like to relax. Some instruction or signal that indicates our state of physical relaxation forms the basis of biofeedback.

Biofeedback helps you regain awareness of the fine changes that occur with relaxation. It makes you aware of the physical sensations that are part of the relaxation response and allows you to find ways to achieve this state at will.

We know that the relaxation state engages the parasympathetic nervous system, which results in a change to our physiology including warming of the skin and increased resistance to electrical conduction as measured by the Galvanic Skin Response. These changes in body function form the basis of the polygraph or lie detector. This is, in a way, biofeedback in reverse. The stress of lying activates the sympathetic nervous system. This produces changes in skin electrical resistance, pulse rate, and blood pressure that are detected by the polygraph.

You can use the same information in learning to relax. The premise is based on the fact that you need some feedback/input to know what it feels like to relax. Instruments measuring temperature, muscle tension, and brain wave activity usually provide this feedback from some monitor or device. This measurement of skin temperature or state of muscle tension is relayed through sound, light, or other means to the person, who then learns and adapts different relaxation techniques to achieve that relaxed state. The instrument allows you to become aware of the physiological changes that occur with relaxation and for you to learn what it takes to produce these changes. When you know what the feeling is, you can tune in to the sensation in your own body that is relaxation and the feedback then becomes internal. Once you learn to do so, you outgrow the need for an external device.

The most common biofeedback techniques involve measuring skin temperature or the degree of muscle tension. Typically, the person is taught basic relaxation methods and is then hooked up to an appropriate monitor, such as a temperature probe taped to a finger. This measures the body's response to relaxation; if relaxation results, skin temperature rises. The person keeps a log of the relaxation methods and the measured response, in this case skin temperature. In this way, the relaxation method that produces the most consistent response is detected. Furthermore, the physical sensation of relaxation starts becoming familiar. The biofeedback instrument provides a bridge to regaining your natural feelings.

Biofeedback instruction is provided by trained professionals and is widely used in pain clinics and headache clinics. Biofeedback is also used to relieve anxiety and counter stress. Typically, weekly biofeedback sessions last forty-five minutes with practice exercises, performed at home, between training sessions. Scientific studies in migraine attest to the effectiveness of relaxation techniques with or without biofeedback. On an average, regular relaxation techniques result in approximately 40 percent fewer headaches. This is similar to the effectiveness of preventive medication.

The Limitations of Biofeedback Therapy

Unfortunately, we have seen that the benefit that many of our patients obtained through biofeedback programs did not last or endure. There are several reasons that limit the use of mechanical devices for relaxation.

- The devices are not very transportable, although small bands (the same principle as a mood ring) that change color with variations in skin temperature can be helpful.
- Some people can learn to change the parameters such as skin temperature without really relaxing.
- Compulsive goal-directed behavior is encouraged by striving to reach the goal, such as changing skin temperature. This can be frustrating and counterproductive. It is hard to let go and relax when a specific task is to be attained.
- There is a danger of the technique becoming mechanical and inflexible where true relaxation should be spontaneously brought about by many different techniques.
- Biofeedback helps as long as the formal course and instruction lasts, but, as we have observed, refresher courses are needed to maintain improvement.
- Some people have difficulty transferring or associating the external indicator on the device with their internal body sensation.
- The relaxation techniques often feel alien and are not easily integrated into daily life, and they are effective only as long as the sessions lasted.

The Closer One Is to Truth, the Simpler Things Become

Over the years I have used biofeedback to complement medical treatments for my patients; I had become increasingly aware of these limitations. There had to be a simpler way to relax: something that does not require instruments, that is flexible and easy to use. In short, I was dissatisfied with the results from standardized electromuscular and thermal biofeedback techniques. The benefit that people had during the course of instruction usually faded away over the ensuing months.

I was seeking a more flexible, less mechanical, and less rigid approach to restore the balance in the autonomic nervous system when I attended one of Dr. Herbert Benson's workshops and was struck by the simplicity of his Relaxation Response. Dr. Benson identified the Relaxation Response and is well known for his work at the Harvard Deaconess mind-body program. Dr. Benson had extensively researched different relaxation methods and had distilled the essence of these techniques. Many Eastern techniques are not suitable for our fast-paced life. The religious-based practices posed a potential conflict with individual religious beliefs. But Dr. Benson found the common thread running through old and ancient meditation and relaxation techniques and gave it scientific validity, naming it the Relaxation Response. This technique, described in his book *The Relaxation Response*, brings the mind and breath together by repeating a phrase or sound to each out-breath. The Relaxation Response then occurs automatically.

The effectiveness and flexibility of these techniques were attractive. If a way is to be found to consistently reduce the effects of stress, it must be uncomplicated, flexible, and enduring. This clicked with me as I recalled a guiding principle: the closer one is to truth, the simpler things become.

Learning to relax at will is the essential first step. All else follows. We based many of the methods in our headache reduction program on the scientific work of Dr. Benson and others. These provide the core of our stress reduction and headache reduction program.

We each use our own internal biofeedback every day. We react to body sensations such as shifting our posture when uncomfortable, clearing our throat, taking a deep breath, or sighing. This, however, is largely unconscious or automatic. We can make this a conscious process, and we can become aware of how our reaction, in turn, changes the sensation.

This "internal" biofeedback is natural and simple, and it does not rely on computers, electronic equipment, or more complicated methods. As we will see in Part II, the techniques can be as simple as learning to watch our breathing.

The Traps and Obstacles in Using Relaxation Techniques

Obstacles—the Real Reasons We Avoid Relaxation

Learning to relax is not easy. How does something so simple become difficult?

The most common reasons we hear in our clinic are related to lack of time and energy. "I have no time." "I have too many things on my plate." "This is not a good time." "I come home from work and I am exhausted." "I will learn to do this when I have more time and energy." When you look at the deeper reasons behind these excuses, you may see several patterns.

Stress Itself
Stress is so pernicious because the state of contraction under stress is often self-perpetuating. When you are in the stress mode, you react and think negatively. If you are in a state of alert you cannot let your guard down without feeling vulnerable. The increased activity of the sympathetic nervous system does not allow for positive thoughts to penetrate, as you remain defensive and on guard. One effect of stress is to reduce your awareness of what you need, including your awareness of the value for self-care. You are in the mode of overactivity and too busy sacrificing yourself for others or your job.

Chronic activation of the sympathetic nervous system consumes your energy and reserve. Little energy is left over if your reacting and self-protection consume you. This withdrawal into yourself is a natural and protective reaction to stress as your energy goes into meeting the challenge or threat. Unless you can find the motivation and awareness to seek periods of relaxation and rest, the cycle of stress will continue. The stress cycle is thus self-perpetuating, leaving you with little time and energy to take countermeasures.

Fear

Fear of letting go of your stress habits is a barrier to learning relaxation methods. The way you defend yourself from stress comes at a high price. These defenses prevent you from feeling the gentle sensations of your own body.

You have come to respect this fear. Many of us just fear being alone—without distractions we have only ourselves. Strange how we come to fear our own company! This is why the effects of chronic stress are undone slowly, at a pace that agrees with and never exceeds your tolerance and comfort. Every person finds his or her own comfort level.

Habit and Inertia

Continued stress becomes a habit. It is hard to change a habit that has become your unconscious way of reacting to the world. Inertia is your resistance to change. In physics, inertia is defined as the resistance of a body at rest to movement. It takes energy to get going. You have seen what chronic stress does to your energy level. It is difficult to learn something new, and you have resistance to work and effort. The paradox here is that work is required in order to rest.

We make it very clear in our classes that the wisdom of the body operates at all levels and that the process of relaxation is self-regulated. There really is nothing to fear but your feelings and sensations. Learning to relax is a gradual process. Your inner wisdom and life restore the balance gradually, peacefully if you begin to remove the obstacles. No one goes beyond his or her level of comfort. There's no goal, no end point. The task is to begin to restore the balance.

Pitfalls

There are several hidden issues that you need to be aware of in using natural relaxation methods to treat your headaches. This is a good time to address these before you embark on the actual exercises in Part II. Here are some of these pitfalls.

Guilt

This is a setup for many migraine sufferers. There are two kinds of headache guilt. You may have experienced guilt in having headaches as well as guilt at getting others down when you cannot function as expected. You feel responsible or at fault for not being able to control these headaches. This negative view is promoted by the prevailing misconception that migraine is a result of your inability to cope or some personality flaw.

If your expectations are unrealistic and you set goals too high, you set yourself up for failure. To restore and maintain your autonomic nervous system balance, you explore different relaxation techniques in order to find what works best for you. It is a trial-and-error process. You do so by assuming some responsibility for your health, but you must be careful not to feel guilty if the techniques are not 100 percent effective. Sometimes these techniques are all you need. At other times they may serve to complement other treatments such as medication.

Some methods may not work for you. Rather than feeling guilty, you move on to explore other methods better suited to your nature and lifestyle. Fear of failure is not a reason to avoid acquiring relaxation skills.

Excessive Striving or Trying Too Hard

Many share what used to be called the migraine personality of being hard-driving type A, goal directed, and successful. You set a goal to relax, reduce stress, and restore balance. There is a risk here that you try too hard and become compulsive about the methods.

This is one of the drawbacks of biofeedback where the goal is set (such as warming our hands) and you strive to achieve it. This hard work can be counterproductive because excessive effort engages the sympathetic nervous system and the stress response rather than its opposite, the Relaxation Response. The paradox here is to achieve the results by "letting go" of the end result. The effort is put into counteracting your tendency to strive hard.

Mysticism

Your ability to relax lies within each of us in what Dr. Cannon called the wisdom of the body. At times, your attunement with your biological core can lead to sensations that are sweet, gentle, and beautiful. The sensations can be so intense that you may find it difficult to accept that they arise from within you. At times like this it is easy to project these feelings outside yourself onto some external source, being, or spirit according to your belief. Whatever your spiritual or religious belief, you can learn to value the precious and gentle sensations within yourself without becoming mystical. Mysticism is a process whereby your inner sensations and wisdom are attributed to some outside source. Your search for connection with the cosmos, spirit, or God is a personal and sacred journey. In our classes, we take care to reassure everyone that sensations arising from contact with your own biological core are life-positive and are consistent with all spiritual and religious beliefs.

Being Impatient

Chronic stress is a habit. It results from years of accumulating stress in the body and mind with chronic activation of the sympathetic nervous system. Over the years you accumulate a stress load. The process of relieving yourself of this burden of heightened sympathetic activity is best done slowly and gradually. Chronic stress causes us to be in a state of contraction or defense. If you relax, let go, and expand too quickly you can feel overwhelmed.

You are not used to the state and may feel vulnerable. This is one of the reasons you fear letting go or losing control.

Gradual restoration of the balance is natural and safe as you slowly begin to adjust the scales and begin to emerge from your protective shell. For some it may feel like gradually emerging from a state of siege to freedom, like a tortoise putting its head out of the shell or a prisoner walking into the sunshine of freedom. There are many inner safeguards that prevent you from moving too quickly in this direction.

Going to Extremes

Just as chronic overactivity of the sympathetic nervous system produces a stress load, the opposite—excessive relaxation—can result from overactivity of the parasympathetic nervous system. The state of balance or health is a dynamic equilibrium of both forces: contraction–expansion, sympathetic–parasympathetic. There is a risk that excessive use of relaxation techniques can make you dull by reducing your vigor and vitality. You do not retreat into these relaxed states to merely withdraw from the world, to avoid issues, or avoid dealing with problems.

Periods of rest and awareness are healthy if followed by action or movement. If you seek to remain in the relaxed state for prolonged periods and use it to avoid activity and responsibility, you risk becoming increasingly passive. This is sometimes the state that mysticism produces, where you long to cloister yourself from the world and achieve a state of quiet peacefulness that nothing can disturb. The balance that you achieve using relaxation techniques is healthy and dynamic and is not one-sided.

You have two ways to try to restore the loss of balance in the body and nervous system. The first, less desirable, option is to reduce the sensitivity of the balance that occurs with increasing stress load and the effect of medication. Alternatively, you can restore your balance by remaining sensitive and aware. Mastery always is evidenced by a light and delicate touch. You can aspire to this! The benefits of being in balance while preserving your sensitivity are seen not only in improved physical well-being and symptom reduction but also in the broadening of perception. By maintaining your sensitive balance, you have a way out of the state of chronic stress that is so often our modern-day trap.

6

Taking Medication to Treat Your Headache

There is, as yet, no perfect treatment for migraine. Despite the discovery of new migraine drugs, there are limits to the use and effectiveness of many medications.

At best, preventive medications are only 40 percent effective in reducing the frequency of headaches, and they all have some side effects. There is now a growing appreciation of problems with overuse of the new migraine-aborting drugs, the triptans. These drugs have changed and revolutionized the treatment of the acute migraine attack. However, recent studies suggest that use of triptan medications for relief of headache should be restricted to no more than two or three times a week. Frequent use of triptans may result in more migraines! Furthermore, regular and frequent use of regular painkillers may cause a worsening of headaches, leading to chronic migraines.

A one-sided approach relying exclusively on medication has its limitations. What are your options? Natural self-care methods enhance the power of medications and reduce your risk of becoming dependent on medications. Careful use of medication is often necessary for control and relief of headache. There is no conflict between using natural relaxation techniques and medication. On the contrary, they complement each other and, in combination, are able to reduce the impact of migraine on your life.

Although you aim, as far as possible, to control your migraines naturally, you may still require medication to control your migraine attacks. Some, particularly those with chronic migraine, will benefit from preventive medication. It is appropriate to relieve the burden of migraine by whatever helpful and healthful means available.

The past decade has witnessed the discovery of powerful new drugs that target the acute migraine attack. By contrast, the development of drugs to *prevent* migraine has lagged behind the acute therapies.

It is estimated that in the United States alone, 150,000 people are disabled by migraine each day! Yet only 10 percent of migraine attacks are treated with the new migraine-specific drugs. There is clearly a discrepancy between the promise of these powerful medications and their actual use and benefit. Why is this so? Based on observation from clinical practice as well as our own migraine experience, we have seen how resistance to taking medication impacts the effectiveness of treatment.

This chapter does not contain a detailed list of the drugs, side effects, or dosages used to treat and prevent migraine headaches. References containing these details are listed in the additional reading at the end of this book.

Drugs to Treat the Acute Migraine Attack

Many of the drugs used to treat and prevent migraine were discovered by chance observation, and for years medical scientists had little idea how they worked. Concepts and theories of migraine were used to explain the action of drugs in migraine. For example, beta-blockers (such as propranolol) were originally developed to treat hypertension and heart disease. In the early trials of these drugs for treatment of hypertension, it was noted that many headache sufferers on this medication reported fewer headaches. This observation led to the testing of the drug in individuals with migraine who had normal blood pressure. This was shown to be effective in reducing the number of headaches.

The beta-blockers soon became accepted treatment for the prevention of migraine. At that time the prevailing theory of migraine was that the headache phase of the migraine attack resulted from dilation of the cranial blood vessels, and the aura, when it occurred, resulted from constriction of the cerebral blood vessels. This was called the vascular theory, and it appeared to fit neatly with the observed phenomena such as the effects of beta-blockers on the blood vessels.

The beta-blockers have an additional and hidden effect in calming down the excitable nerve cells in that part of the brain that generates the migraine. This is how they prevent migraine.

Drugs known as ergotamines or ergot alkaloids (which were derived from a fungus that grows on rye) had been known since the 1940s to be effective in stopping a migraine attack. These ergot drugs constrict the blood vessels and appeared to be another perfect fit with the then prevailing theory that migraines were due to changes in blood vessel caliber. We now know that the change in the caliber and diameter of the blood vessels is part, but not the primary event, of the migraine attack.

The ergot drugs are also now known to act on certain chemical receptors on the nerve endings where they reduce the release of inflammatory-causing chemicals onto the blood vessels. The property of ergotamines to constrict the blood vessel—initially thought to be the primary action of the drug in migraine—now becomes an unwanted effect and accounts for the major side effects of these drugs. In the Middle Ages, contamination of rye with the ergot fungus caused epidemics of ergot poisoning called Saint Anthony's fire. This condition included symptoms of psychosis and loss of limbs from gangrene. It is interesting to note that the early drugs to treat migraine were derived from a poison.

With the transition from the vascular theory of migraine to the neuronal theory, we have developed a greater understanding of how the drugs work. This understanding and years of research led to the astonishing breakthrough in the early 1990s of the first migraine designer drug—sumatriptan. This heralded a new era in the treatment of acute migraine attacks. Sumatriptan was the first of a class of drugs called the triptans. Triptans act on the nerve endings by activating a specific inhibitory chemical receptor. This action shuts off a migraine attack by preventing the release of inflammatory-causing chemicals from the nerve endings onto the blood vessels. The same chemical receptors are also found on the blood vessels in the scalp, outside the brain but within the skull, and, to a lesser degree, on the coronary blood vessels.

Since the development of sumatriptan (Imitrex), other triptans have been developed and marketed for use in migraine. These include zolmitriptan (Zomig), rizatriptan (Maxalt), naratriptan (Amerge), almotriptan (Axert), and eletriptan (Relpax), with several more in development. These triptans are all similar in effectiveness but differ slightly in formulation, absorption, and tolerability.

For the first time, a class of migraine drugs has been developed based on the understanding of the chemistry of migraine rather than trying to fit observations into prevailing theory. This is a wonderful application of the scientific method, and it has revolutionized the medical treatment of the acute migraine attack.

Yet the triptans are not perfect. We do not understand why these drugs work in only 80 percent of migraines. They have potential side effects, and they have to be used under medical supervision. The triptans are mostly short-acting with the result that the headache may come back once the drug wears off. Nevertheless, these drugs are a significant advance and have helped many migraine sufferers, as one person described it, to "get my life back."

Removing the fear and anticipation of your next uncontrolled headache is a cornerstone of migraine treatment. This allows you the freedom to make arrangements, work, or socialize without the fear of having an uncontrolled headache and letting others down. Taking other factors into consideration, the triptans often form the center of drug treatment of migraine around which other treatments are planned.

Drugs to Relieve the Pain of Migraine

Over-the-Counter Nonprescription
Acetaminophen
Aspirin
Nonsteroidals: ibuprofen, naproxen
Combination with caffeine: Excedrin, Anacin

Prescription
Nonsteroidals
Ergotamine tartrate (Cafergot, Ergostat)
Dihydroergotamine (DHE, Migranal)
Triptans: sumatriptan (Imitrex), zolmitriptan (Zomig),
      rizatriptan (Maxalt), naratriptan (Amerge), almotriptan
      (Axert), eletriptan (Relpax)
Painkillers with butabarbital: Fiorinal, Fioricet, Esgic
Opiates, narcotics: codeine, hydrocodone, propoxyphene,
      oxycodone

Not all migraine requires prescription medication. Over-the-counter painkillers such as aspirin, ibuprofen, naproxen, and painkillers combined with caffeine are often helpful if taken early on for the less severe migraines. A 1998 study shows that the use of over-the-counter pain medication for migraine has remained essentially unchanged in the past decade, with approximately 57 percent of migraine sufferers using over-the-counter medications exclusively. But self-medication often has limited effectiveness.

All medications taken for migraine attack are more effective when taken early. When the triptans were initially introduced, they were suggested as treatment of last resort and reserved only for a severe or uncontrolled migraine attack. This was called a "step care" approach, using the weaker treatments initially and then, as these failed to control the headache, moving on to more effective medication. This recommendation changed as the benefits from their use earlier in the migraine attack became apparent. The triptan drugs are best used early in an attack, and you don't have to wait for a weaker medication to fail first. Based on experience, you usually know at the onset of a headache whether a simple or nonprescription painkiller will work.

Medication to Prevent Migraine

Basically, preventive medicines raise the threshold for getting a migraine. These drugs work in different ways to stabilize the excitable nerve cells that generate the migraine. The development of specific preventive medication for migraine lags behind that of the acute treatments such as the triptans by at least a decade or more. All the drugs used to prevent migraine [except for methysergide (Sansert) which was developed in the 1960s] were developed for treatment of other medical conditions. We have no new medications specifically designed to prevent migraine headaches.

Preventive treatment of migraine with medication is considered when:

- Migraine attacks are of sufficient frequency and severity to adversely affect quality of life
- Migraine attacks continue to be disabling despite acute treatment

Drugs to Prevent Migraine

Antiseizure Drugs
Divalproex sodium (Depakote)
Gabapentin (Neurontin)
Topiramate (Topamax)

Antidepressants
Amitriptyline (Elavil)
Fluoxetine (Prozac)

Beta-blockers
Propranolol (Inderal)
Atenolol, timolol

Calcium Channel Blockers
Verapamil
Diltiazem

Nonsteroidals
Aspirin
Naproxen

Serotonin Antagonists
Methysergide (Sansert)
Cyproheptadine (Periactin)

- The frequency of migraines is so great that there is a risk of overuse of acute therapies
- Acute treatments cannot be used because of other medical considerations

Like the beta-blockers, most drugs used to prevent or decrease the number of migraine headaches were discovered by clinical or accidental observation. There is still much misconception about these drugs.

Certain antidepressants that belong to a class of tricyclics (including amitriptyline) are known to decrease migraine frequency. These medications help prevent migraine when used in low doses—too low to have any antidepressant effect. Like the beta-blockers, the effect of these medications in preventing headache is an unintended benefit. These medications have been used since the 1970s to treat migraine even when there is no depression. These drugs do *not* prevent migraine by treating depression. They stabilize the excitable nerve cells in the part of the brain that generates the migraine. They do so by down-regulating or reducing certain chemical receptors on the surface of the nerve cells. When the words *headache* and *antidepressant* appear on the same page, it is erroneously assumed that the headache is caused by depression.

As the focus shifts to finding ways to reduce the excitability of nerve cells thought to be the biological basis of migraine, attention is turning to drugs that have this effect—specifically the antiseizure medications. All the antiseizure drugs, by one mechanism of action or another, act by reducing the excitability of nerve cells. A seizure is caused by the spread of uncontained and abnormal electrical discharge produced by groups of nerve cells that discharge in an abnormal or uninhibited way. The antiseizure drugs thus prevent and contain this abnormal overactivity of nerve cells.

Migraine and seizures are two distinctly different disorders. Yet they are similar in that they are both paroxysmal disorders, which means that they both produce "attacks" of a disorder—a migraine in the one and a seizure in the other. These attacks are caused by a discharge of excitable nerve cells. This is where the similarity ends. In migraine, this neural discharge leads not to buildup of electrical discharge in the brain (as occurs in a seizure) but to changes in brain chemistry and blood vessel caliber.

The first of the antiseizure medications to be approved for migraine prevention, and meet the FDA requirements, was divalproex sodium (Depakote). Other medications in this class are currently under investigation and hold promise for future treatment.

The Special Problem of Chronic Migraine and Analgesic Use

For some, migraine is a progressive disorder. We do not yet understand what causes this progression and what the risk factors are. Chronic migraine sufferers often begin having migraine in their teens or twenties. The migraines gradually become more frequent, evolving to daily or almost daily headache. The daily headache is less intense than a full migraine, but full migraine attacks are superimposed on this low-grade everyday headache. This type of headache is defined by the International Headache Society as a headache at least 50 percent of the time or fifteen days out of a month. People with this headache pattern, called chronic migraine or transformed migraine, comprise 4 to 5 percent of the general population but make up approximately 80 percent of those who are seen at specialty headache clinics.

This group of headache sufferers most commonly gets into trouble with overusing painkillers and developing Analgesic Rebound syndrome (see page 103). Chronic migraine sufferers more commonly have other comorbid conditions such as irritable bowel syndrome, fibromyalgia, depression, anxiety, and panic disorder. Because they use medications more frequently, there's a greater occurrence of side effects from painkillers such as stomach upset or ulcers.

There are several factors that predispose one to this pattern of chronic migraine. A genetic predisposition is evidenced by the fact that 80 percent of chronic daily headache sufferers have a family history of headache medication overuse. Other factors that increase the probability of developing chronic migraine include an imbalance in neurotransmitter chemical levels in the brain resulting from accumulating stress on the nervous system as well as emotional stress and physical trauma. This pattern again indicates the sensitivity and vulnerability of the nervous system in migraine.

Analgesic Overuse and Rebound Syndrome

Analgesic Rebound syndrome is a problem unique to migraine! We think of it as a faulty "off switch." With analgesic overuse, the part of the brain that switches off a migraine begins to fail. It becomes harder to turn off those nerve cells that are overactive during a migraine headache.

When you begin using more and more painkillers to suppress the headache, the brain mechanism for switching off the headache starts shutting down and relief of pain becomes dependent on the painkiller. The intrinsic pain suppression system, which is already faulty, starts closing up shop. The receptors on the nerve cells that are responsible for stopping pain begin to disappear. This has been documented in animal experiments. When the painkiller wears off, the headache returns—often worse than before. This is known as rebound. You need another painkiller to relieve the pain and eventually a cycle of growing dependency develops. Also, tolerance to the painkillers develops over time, so more and stronger medications are needed to get the same relief. Another unintended effect of this vicious cycle of pain–painkiller–pain is that the frequent use of painkillers blocks or interferes with the effectiveness of medications given to prevent headache. Studies have shown that it takes up to six to twelve weeks (or longer) off all painkillers before you regain your ability to switch off a headache naturally.

Dr. K. Michael Welch's research group at the University of Kansas has demonstrated very subtle changes in the pain control part of the brain in people with chronic migraine. These researchers used techniques of nuclear magnetic resonance spectroscopy (which can noninvasively measure certain chemicals in the brain). They observed an increase in the deposition of iron pigment in this part of the brain. The degree of nerve cell damage and iron pigment deposition is greatest in chronic migraine sufferers. Dr. Welch's research provides the first evidence of permanent chemical change in the brain in chronic migraine sufferers. There are several theories to account for this observation. We accept the view that this represents the burden of oxidation stress—affecting that part of the brain that has been excessively stressed and is most vulnerable. It is as though the intrinsic pain suppression system becomes burned out or exhausted.

How to Determine If You Are Taking Too Many Painkillers

The improvement in headache following withdrawal of painkillers is the only certain way to make a diagnosis of analgesic rebound or medication overuse headache. There are, however, some guidelines that indicate a high probability of medication overuse headache. The International Headache Society recently defined these guidelines.

These guidelines indicate how vulnerable many migraine sufferers are to the development of rebound and analgesic dependency. Analgesic rebound is unique to migraine and does not occur in other chronic pain conditions such as back pain or arthritis.

Treatment of rebound headaches usually requires a specialist, lots of education, and a caring treatment partnership with combined use of painkiller withdrawal, preventive medication, and relaxation techniques.

Chronic daily headaches are very stressful. The cycle of pain and stress is ongoing and the whole nervous system becomes sensitized to pain. The sufferer is in a chronic stress mode, always warding off and anticipating the next headache. This is why the World Health Organization ranks chronic migraine as one of the most disabling medical conditions!

Criteria for Medication Overuse Headache

Headaches on more than fifteen days per month.
Painkillers required for two or more days per week (depending on the substance) for more than one month.

Criteria for overuse of triptans include use of any triptan drug on a regular basis for more than three days a week for at least two weeks.

Criteria for overuse of simple painkillers include three or more tablets per day regularly for more than four days each week.

Criteria for overuse of painkillers containing barbiturates (such as Fiorinal, Fioricet, etc.) include two or more tablets each day regularly for more than three days per week.

Criteria for overuse of opioid analgesics (narcotic drugs containing codeine, hydrocodone, oxycodone) include use of these medications more than two days each week on a regular basis.

The Limitations of Drug Treatment
There is always a downside to using medication, and drugs used to relieve and prevent migraine are no exception.

Issues of Preventive Treatment
Side Effects
The ability of certain drugs to prevent migraine was first discovered by chance observation. Most of the medications used to prevent migraine were discovered when patients taking the medications for high blood pressure or seizures reported having fewer headaches. The medications were then tested on people who had migraine.

Only a few drugs have FDA approval as migraine preventives.

Most of the medications used in medical practices to prevent migraine, although effective, have never been fully tested for that use.

All drugs, even aspirin, have potential side effects. A side effect is an undesirable, unwanted action of the medication. It is the risk or price to pay to obtain the desired effect of the drug. Side effects vary according to the type of medication, dosage, and sensitivity to medication. It is this individual sensitivity that causes so many migraine sufferers to experience difficulties with daily medication. This sensitivity to medication is another aspect of the enhanced responsiveness that is part and parcel of the migraine trait. Most headache specialists recognize this sensitivity in prescribing medication for migraine.

Currently we have no way to accurately predict what class of medication will work and for whom, although there are helpful guidelines and principles based on scientific studies. On average, it takes a trial of three or four different medications in different doses before an effective tolerable medication is found to reduce migraine. This trial and error is required because different classes of drugs act by different chemical mechanisms and individuals react differently to each.

Sometimes a medication works by reducing a specific chemical receptor on the nerve cell that makes the cell less reactive. Other times the excitability of the nerve cells is reduced by increasing an inhibitory chemical in the brain called GABA (gamma amino butyric acid). These drugs have different mechanisms of action but they have the same end result of raising the migraine threshold, stabilizing the nerve cells, and making it harder to get a migraine no matter what the trigger.

It takes so many trials of medication to find the "best" medication due to the side effects. This sensitivity to medication is largely seen in the occurrence of sedation, weight gain, mood changes, and diminished energy level. This is not an allergy but rather sensitivity to the effects of chemicals on the nervous system. Many migraine sufferers are sensitive to the effects of other chemicals, such as alcohol, which is a central nervous system depressant drug. Even if the alcohol does not trigger headache, migraine-prone individuals often become sleepy and feel dull with small amounts of alcohol.

Doctors who are not used to treating migraine sufferers often become frustrated by their patients' intolerance to medications, particularly if they don't realize that very small doses of medication have to be used. Physicians often prescribe medication in a "therapeutic" rather than minimal dose. The treatment of migraine is different from most other medical conditions in which medication is administered in a curative or effective dose.

What Drugs Cannot Do

Most medications that reduce the enhanced responsiveness of the nervous system do so by dampening down and reducing sympathetic tone—that is, they reduce the tendency to the fight-or-flight response. The trade-off is a dulling of the nervous system. What actually happens in the state of heightened responsiveness is a loss of balance between the sympathetic and parasympathetic systems. In "overdrive," stress, or in response to pain, the sympathetic part of the nervous system is activated. The restoration of the balance can be attempted pharmacologically by reducing the sympathetic overdrive.

The following story illustrates this. Terri, a fifty-six-year-old female with a long history of migraine and heightened stress responsiveness, has responded to Prozac. This has resulted in a reduction in anxiety and a modest decrease in headache frequency, but she feels that this is a superficial phenomenon. She describes feeling dull on the surface but still in turmoil underneath. This is sensed as a feeling of restlessness and heightened stress responsiveness with a dull exterior. Although calm on the surface, she has not attained a sense of peace; although functioning better, she still experiences a sense of unease.

We have no drugs to activate the parasympathetic response or to induce the relaxation response. All tranquilizer drugs reduce the sympathetic tone of the sympathetic nervous system and the response is entirely dependent on the drug. Once the drug is discontinued, a rebound state of heightened responsiveness or anxiety is often experienced.

The relaxation response has to happen from within and cannot be imposed from without. It involves essentially a letting go, to which the body responds with restoration of balance. This is done spontaneously and occurs without taking conscious thought and is not maintained by effort of will. That is, unlike a drug effect, its benefit extends far beyond the administration of treatment—in this case, the ultimate benefit is relaxation.

Natural relaxation results in a sense of well-being and sharpened or heightened perception—the opposite of the dampening effect of drugs. Enhanced responsiveness of the nervous system significantly contributes to the misery of migraine. It must be recognized and treated with respect. In our view, the suppression of vitality is the main drawback to the exclusive reliance on medication for the prevention of migraine.

Effectiveness of Medication
At best, the preventive medications are effective only approximately 40 percent of the time. For example, studies on divalproex sodium (Depakote), which meets FDA approval as a migraine preventive drug, show that 43 to 50 percent of patients have greater than 50 percent reduction in headache frequency. About 20 percent of patients discontinued therapy because of their inability to tolerate the medication. Statistics for other preventive medications are similar, at only about 40 percent effectiveness.

Although not perfect, these medication are an enormous help in preventing headaches in someone who has frequent and disabling migraine. The difference in coping with one migraine each week compared to every other day is enormous! All these medications are helpful and we prescribe the whole range of medications in our practice for migraine prevention. The downside to these medications, however, must be appreciated and factored into their use.

It Takes Time

The other problem with preventive medications is the delay in assessing effectiveness. Preventive medications can take weeks or even months to become effective. It takes time for the hyperexcitability of the nerve cells to be calmed and chemical changes in the brain to become stabilized. Many people do not appreciate this and end up discarding their preventive medications after the first two or three weeks. In reality, an adequate trial of preventive medication takes approximately two to three months!

This is one reason that patience and persistence are so important. Occasionally we'll see someone who seeks help for his or her headaches and presents a long laundry list of failed treatments. It is quite a task to analyze the failed treatments. Sometimes the treatment failed because the dose of the drug was too high or side effects were experienced. At other times, the medication was not given a fair trial and was stopped after only a few weeks. Also, the use of daily painkillers blocks the preventive drugs from working. Medication failure leads to increasing frustration and growing pessimism.

Partnership

Finding the right medication is not easy. This is why a patient-caregiver partnership is so vital. The physician and the migraine sufferer form a therapeutic alliance. This partnership is based on trust, education, support, and patience. It is time-consuming but necessary. The migraine sufferer learns to be patient and trust in the process, knowing that he or she will be heard if there's a problem with medication. The physician also exercises patience and learns to be tolerant of his or her own frustration in dealing with patients who are discouraged and overwhelmed.

Many chronic migraine patients are considered "needy." They can sense the physician's frustration each time they report on a new problem with their medication, even minor symptoms such as dry mouth. This is one reason why there are so many "lapsed consulters"—people who once consulted a doctor for migraine but no longer do so.

Still, there have been considerable advances in understanding the treatment of migraine. Two large migraine studies showed that the number of lapsed consulters dropped from 50 percent in 1989 to 21 percent in 1999. This is a move in the right direction and gives us hope for the future as it shows a trend to better understanding and more treatment options.

Coexisting Conditions

As mentioned in chapter 2, the migraine sufferer may have other coexisting but unrelated medical disorders. The selection of medication is colored by the presence of these associated conditions. For example, someone who has mild hypertension and migraine may have both conditions improved with a beta-blocker or calcium channel blocker, which has an effect on separate and unrelated disorders. By contrast, beta-blockers cannot be used in someone who has asthma because these drugs can worsen an asthmatic condition.

So, not only is the migraine sufferer more sensitive to the effects of medication, but the presence of associated or comorbid conditions may limit what medications can be used. Ignoring the coexisting condition adds to the risk of untoward side effects and an unsatisfactory outcome on medication.

Issues of Acute Treatments

The new class of migraine drugs, the triptans, have revolutionized the treatment of the acute migraine attack. Despite the effectiveness of these medications, there are still problems with the drug treatment of the acute migraine attack.

Access to Treatment

If migraine is not medically diagnosed, there can obviously be no prescribed treatment. In a 1999 survey, 52 percent of migraine sufferers in the United States had no medical diagnosis. There are barriers to the diagnosis of migraine including bias, prejudice, lack of knowledge, and negative prior medical experiences that lead many migraine sufferers to rely solely on over-the-counter painkillers and self-medication. The same survey found that 57 percent of migraine sufferers in the United States rely exclusively on over-the-counter painkillers. While this is helpful for the most part, we know that self-medication fails in many cases. What then? A visit to the emergency room or a lost day from work!

The statistics attest to the fact that most migraines are not adequately treated. From the 1999 Second American Migraine Study, 53 percent of migraine sufferers reported requiring bed rest or experienced severe impairment of function, and 39 percent stated they were somewhat impaired. A full 91 percent reported not being able to function effectively at work during the migraine attack! This is another indication that most migraine attacks are not adequately treated.

Attitudes toward Treating Migraine

Physician Attitudes

From 1989 to 1999, the number of migraine sufferers seeking medical help increased, but a much smaller increase was noted in those taking prescription medications. This again indicates that, despite medical consultation, most migraine is still not adequately treated. Reluctance to accept migraine as a "real" or legitimate medical disorder still stands in the way of adequate recognition and treatment.

Migraine is still not considered a serious or legitimate medical disorder by many doctors despite the overwhelming evidence of disability and erosion of quality of life in migraine. Migraine sufferers may actually perpetuate this shortcoming. Headache patients often minimize their suffering in reporting their headaches to their doctors and often doctors do not ask about disability. Memory of pain fades and is suppressed; hence, reporting of headache is minimized. "I don't recall details of the headache I had three weeks ago, and it does not seem so bad now that I'm feeling well."

The attitude and receptivity of the treating physician are important. Your doctor is more likely to prescribe medication for migraine if he or she appreciates the degree of disability and sickness that accompanies your headache. We wonder if the prescribing habits of physicians who are themselves migraine sufferers differ from their nonmigraineur colleagues.

The Attitude of the Migraine Sufferer

Expectations

Your expectations of medication can sometimes be too high. If you experience incomplete relief from the pain, you may feel disillusioned and give up.

A 1998 survey by Drs. Richard Lipton and Walter Stewart showed that

- Twenty-nine percent of migraine sufferers were very satisfied with the treatment for acute attacks.

Of those not satisfied with treatment:

- Eighty-seven percent found that pain relief took too long.
- Eighty-four percent found that not all their pain was relieved.

- In 84 percent the medication did not always work.
- In 71 percent the headache returned.
- Thirty-five percent experienced side effects.

These statistics show that there are limitations to medication in the treatment of migraine. This may also make you more realistic in your expectations. It also indicates room for improvement, and we must look for ways to improve treatment results while we wait for the development of new drugs. One way we can do this, as we shall see in chapter 7, is to use relaxation techniques to enhance the effectiveness of medication.

Resistance and Delay in Taking Medication

In another 1998 study of emotion and attitudes in taking medication for migraine attack, only three out of forty-four persons stated that their mood was not influenced by the attack. The others reported various emotions ranging from despair, fear, panic, and helplessness. Depression was the most commonly recalled emotion. In the study 75 percent expressed an ambivalent or negative attitude to their medication. One-third reported they tried to avoid taking their medication if at all possible. Only 23 percent reported a positive attitude to taking their medication. A further item of interest is that the main reason most people take medication is for relief of pain (57 percent), but 43 percent do not expect to get rid of the pain. They just want to be able to function. The expectation is very low, and they just want to get by for the rest of the day and not have to leave work or give up their obligations.

The delay in taking medication in a migraine attack reduces the effectiveness. A delay results in less pain relief and a greater chance that the headache will recur. There are several reasons why you may delay taking medication for migraine attack, and it is important to address them.

Attitude and Emotion
The predominant mood upon getting another headache is depression. This feeling of despair is coupled with denial.

> "This is not another headache."
> "I cannot believe I am getting another headache."
> "I cannot deal with this."
> "I will wait this out. Maybe it will go away."

These frequently expressed sentiments show how you may try to will the headache away or deny that it's coming on. Unfortunately, it does not help.

Use of relaxation exercises coupled with a shift in attitude can make all the difference to successful control of the migraine attack. Viewing the headache as a cue for self-care helps change things. Chapter 7 is devoted to this aspect of managing the acute headache storm.

This shift from a stress-reacting to a life-supporting response can make an unbelievable difference. Seeing your medication as a gift helps engender a positive attitude. Understanding that you can take action as the headache storm approaches replaces your feelings of passivity and hopelessness with action.

Fearing Loss of Efficacy
Yet another commonly expressed reason for delaying headache treatment is the experience that repeated use of painkillers often leads to tolerance and loss of effectiveness. More frequent doses and stronger medications are required to obtain the same effect. "Once aspirin used to work. Now I need prescription painkillers" is a frequently heard experience.

The new migraine drugs—mostly the triptans—do not exhibit this phenomenon of tolerance. Studies have shown that the triptan drugs do not become less effective with repeated use over time. Realizing this should make you less reluctant to take prescription medication when necessary.

How Do I Know It Is a Migraine?

This is a difficult problem, as most migraine sufferers also experience other headache types as well. You do not want to use your precious prescription migraine medication if it is not a migraine. "You don't use an elephant gun to shoot a gnat," one of my mentors used to say.

Many people "screen" their headaches with over-the-counter painkillers at the onset of the headache if they are not sure it is a migraine. If the medication does not work, then their prescription drug is used.

One of the benefits of practicing relaxation techniques at the onset of a headache is the awareness that relaxation creates. You become finely aware of what is happening in your body. You tune in to the subtle signals of a migraine: signals you so often override and ignore, including light sensitivity, feeling chilled, slight waves of nausea, or other particular cues. Once you are aware of these signals, you will know what action to take—with or without medication.

Hoarding

No headache sufferer should be without the means for acute relief. Yet some headache sufferers deny themselves treatment in order to keep a supply of medication on hand. Some of the prescription migraine drugs (particularly the triptans) are expensive and pharmaceutical plans often approve only limited quantities of the drug on a monthly basis. "This stuff is like gold to me. I will keep it and use it only when I have to."

This is a rationing of effective medical treatment. Many feel it is preferable to suffer a migraine now than having no medication for the next headache. Being without effective medication adds to the anticipatory stress of migraine. Running out of medication deprives the migraine sufferer of choosing which particular migraine to treat. You should have sufficient medication available for the relief of each headache until the headache frequency can be reduced through preventive measures.

Fear of Side Effects

No treatment, as we have seen, is free of side effects. It is important for you to be informed about your medication and its potential benefits and risks. When used according to medical guidelines (particularly avoiding the ergotamines and triptans in the presence of coronary artery disease), the drugs are safe and effective. A trial of one or several medications may be needed to determine which works best and with the least side effects. Here, again, a close therapeutic partnership with the physician is necessary.

A mail survey study found that two-thirds of migraine sufferers delayed or avoided taking a prescription medication for fear of side effects. This led to delay in treatment in 23 percent and avoiding treatment in 44 percent of migraine episodes in the six months preceding the survey.

The fear of side effects has to be addressed with your doctor. Some of these drugs have to be used with caution since they have rarely been reported to produce coronary spasm in people who have coronary artery disease. However, the very small risk of taking the drug should be balanced against suffering repeated disabling migraine attacks. To put this in perspective, a study of twelve thousand patients taking triptan medication for migraine, including injectable sumatriptan, found no significant adverse cardiovascular effects.

Although we have no definitive studies, observation from clinical practice leads us to believe that many of the potential side effects are reduced when the treatment is taken when the headache sufferer is in the relaxed state. This is an additional reason why relaxation is part of the prescription. Think of this for a moment. A shift in attitude and decreased tone of the sympathetic nervous system not only improve effectiveness of treatment but also reduce the risk of adverse reactions.

The Stress Reaction

When you anticipate pain, you engage the fight-or-flight stress response. You tense your muscles and constrict the blood vessels in your extremities as you try to ward off the migraine. This often worsens the headache by increasing muscle tightness, elevating blood pressure and pulse rate. You also reduce your breathing. We have heard it more than once: "I am even afraid to breathe when I feel a migraine coming on." This stress reaction is automatic. You take your medication and then anxiously and tensely wait for the drug to work.

Many migraine sufferers know that their medications are more effective if they can rest or relax for a short while. The migraine pain and sickness come in waves. With each crescendo you tighten up, brace yourself. You are afraid to let go as the pain and sickness become more intense.

Relaxation techniques improve and hasten the effectiveness of medication and provide you a measure of control over what is happening in your body. Dr. Ferdinand Lamaze used the principles of breathing into the pain to ride with the waves of discomfort in devising the exercises that bear his name to help women in labor. You can use similar ways to deliver yourself from your headaches. Instead of fighting a migraine with tense muscles and a negative attitude, you can engage the wisdom of your body to help control pain and improve the outcome and effectiveness of medication. You can learn to be kind and gentle to yourself when you need it the most.

New and potent migraine-specific drugs continue to evolve from understanding the biology of migraine. The introduction of the triptan drugs in the past twelve years has dramatically improved the treatment of the acute migraine attack. Sadly, the development of safe and specific migraine preventive treatment is still years away. Yet, despite these advances in medication and the availability of effective powerful drugs, studies clearly show that medication alone is not the answer. Treatment is still underutilized, underprescribed, and avoided for fear of side effects.

The barriers to more effective treatments can be removed if we understand our resistance to treatment, address our fears, and respect our health.

The migraine trait is innate and biologically determined. You have to learn to live with your tendency to have headaches. You can do this by respecting your vulnerability and using whatever means you have to control the attacks and prevent them from occurring.

Migraine is a thief! It is a medical disorder that would steal your joy, vitality, and productivity. You do not have to limit yourself to only one form of treatment—you have many options. Drug and natural or nondrug treatments give you flexibility and are mutually synergistic. Relaxation techniques and medication are not mutually exclusive. Blending of timeless inner wisdom with newer technologies is a powerful combination in controlling migraine!

PART II

HARP:
The Headache
Reduction Program

The Headache Reduction Program

Dear Donna and Dr. Livingstone,
This is a note of thanks for the gentle lessons you shared throughout our classes together. I have continued to put into practice the techniques that I have learned and remain headache free. There have been days when a headache was imminent, but I have employed the Relaxation Response and taken pain medication when needed with positive results. The worst symptom of migraine has been extreme fatigue, for which a long nap or early to bed has helped.

I think the clearest point made for me was a more complete understanding of the Relaxation Response and the need for daily "vacations" into relaxation and mindfulness. I've learned that it does not work as a quick fix when everything else has failed and the body has not made relaxation a routine to begin with. Also, that it is not one more way to achieve a higher goal, but in fact a letting go of goals and objectives for a sustained period of time daily.

Many, many thanks for a well-run class, fond memories, and tools for better living!

Sincerely,
Lorrie

Lorrie came to the Princeton Headache Clinic with a long history of migraines. She had heard about the positive health benefits of stress management but was unsure how to integrate relaxation into her busy life. Her letter describes how the Headache Reduction Program (HARP) helped her gain control of headaches in two key ways.

First, she is more in tune to her early migraine signals and takes action before the headache becomes severe. She has learned the self-care skills of using the Relaxation Response, taking her pain medication when necessary at the onset of the headache, and resting up when she feels fatigued.

Second, Lorrie has learned to prevent headaches by making relaxation a routine part of life. She takes daily "vacations" from the pressures of goals and objectives, with periods of meditation and mindfulness. These are the "tools for better living" we present in Part II of *Breaking the Headache Cycle*.

Starting with Stress Awareness

The first step of the program involves personal awareness of stress. Look at your headaches as one way that your body signals that something's wrong—a signal to stop and ask, What's going on in my life? What kinds of stress am I under? Is there a balance in my life between work and rest/recreation? Am I taking good care of myself?

At the Princeton Headache Clinic, we ask patients the same types of questions. We often hear, "Oh, I'm not stressed, I like my job, I spend a lot of hours at it, but it's something I like to do. I don't even get headaches during the week as often as the weekends." Or some people say, "Let's get real. I don't have any time for relaxation. I have a lot of responsibilities (as a parent, spouse, student, or employee) that I just can't get rid of. So I just have to live with stress. There's nothing I can do about it." Although stress may be inevitable, there are practical and effective ways to counteract stress. The HARP program will teach you how to balance out the stress in your life with relaxation techniques.

Start by asking yourself if you are operating under any of the following misconceptions:

1. *If I'm happy and stimulated by my life, then I can't be suffering from stress.*

Even when we love our jobs and our families, they still involve plenty of demands and the need to adapt and respond actively, which is another way to define stress.

2. *If stress is triggering my headaches, then wouldn't I be getting headaches only when I'm under the most stress?*

Migraine headaches can be triggered by changes in stress levels, both up and down. If stress levels are up all week without periods of relaxation, then the downtime on weekends or vacations can trigger post-stress headaches.

3. *There's no way I can find the time to relax every day. It just isn't realistic in this busy, competitive world.*

Relaxation does not have to involve long periods of time. Even one or two minutes of focused attention on breathing can produce the beneficial physiologic and mental changes associated with the Relaxation Response. Even the most skeptical people find small periods of time during the day—while commuting to work, walking the dog, or waiting in line at the grocery store—where they can start to make a habit of mindful relaxation. Plus, studies show that work efficiency decreases when stress levels climb too high. Short breaks enhance your performance and efficiency, which makes up for the time you spent relaxing.

4. *I don't see how relaxation can help my headaches—they are usually triggered by changes in the weather and things that are not under my control.*

The HARP techniques help control headaches in two ways. They help relieve the pain of a migraine when it occurs, and, when practiced regularly, they raise your threshold for migraine, making you more headache resistant no matter what the triggers.

5. *Since stress is unavoidable, I have no choice but to live with it, grin and bear it.*

Although many of the stressors in your life may be out of your control, your perception of these stressors and your response to them *are* in your control. In Western culture, people are often driven by the goals they wish to accomplish, and their last priority is care of the self. When they finally give themselves time to relax, during vacations or weekends or in retirement, it can be difficult to do. Think about what you did last weekend. Is your "free" time filled with tasks and appointments and scheduled activities, with little time to yourself for kicking back and simply relaxing? In the words of one clinic patient, "I thought when I retired, I could relax and feel less edgy and keyed up. I thought I would have fewer headaches. But I feel the same. I still make lists of everything I have to do that day, and get upset if I don't accomplish each one."

You need to learn how to relax, how to let go of goals and worries and concerns for a period of time each day. That's what you will learn through HARP, how to use skills like focused breathing, meditation, and stretching to make relaxation a regularly practiced health habit.

Using the HARP Techniques

The following story illustrates how a person who is dealing with an oncoming headache uses relaxation techniques to gain control of the situation. Maryann is going on a camping vacation with her husband and three children. After packing the family's gear all evening (and into the night), she sits in the passenger seat of the car as they motor up to the mountains at 6 A.M. Finding the glare of the sunrise painful, Maryann closes her eyes and feels the familiar tightening in the back of her head and the dull feeling of pressure across her forehead, settling above her left temple. She skipped breakfast and now feels slightly irritable and hungry. "No, I can't believe I'm getting a headache," she moans to herself. Almost immediately, the negative thoughts begin: "I was such an idiot not to prepare all week. As usual I waited until the day before, and of course no one else lifted a finger to help. Why is it always my responsibility? I don't even like camping! And now I'm getting another headache that will probably last all week. If it gets bad, I'm going to get carsick, and my family is going to hate me. These headaches are always ruining everybody's fun."

Fortunately, Maryann has taken the Headache Reduction Program. She recognizes her stress response and the signs that a migraine is under way. She recalls what she learned—first focus on the breath. She takes a deep breath in, lets it out with an audible sigh, then loosens the tension in her abdomen and lets herself breathe fully. "I see I'm getting stressed out. This won't help. I've got to let it go." She becomes aware of tension in her body, uncrosses her legs, settles back in her seat, loosens the tension in her face, jaw, shoulders, the places she knows reflexively tighten in response to stress and pain. She breathes in to the tight places, breathes out the tension.

Feeling more relaxed and in control with every breath, she replaces the negative thoughts with more constructive self-talk, "OK, I can handle this. I've had many headaches before and I can deal with them. They don't last forever. Right now I need to relax and take care of myself. I'll take my pain reliever now. It will work faster. Just rest and remember how well the medicine works for me. I'll feel better soon." She tells her family, "Hold on, I'm getting a migraine." That's their cue to dampen the noise and clatter and give her time out to relax and breathe, so she can recover as quickly as possible. Within an hour, Maryann feels her headache fading away.

Later that day, while marking this headache in her headache diary, she asks herself, What triggered that one? Without using it as an occasion for self-blame, she uses her headaches as something to learn from. She knows pretrip preparations are a big stressor and plans to talk with her family about working together and getting prepared a bit earlier. She promises to get a good night's sleep before a trip and not skip breakfast, even if it means leaving the house a little later than planned.

Maryann congratulates herself for coping so effectively with her headache. She used the opportunity to take care of her needs. She tuned in to the anger, frustration, and tension that were mounting inside her, and she countered them with her focused attention to rhythmic diaphragmatic breathing and release of muscle tension. She didn't hesitate to take her analgesic at the headache's onset, when she recognized her personal migraine warning signals of irritability and light sensitivity. She feels more committed than ever to her daily practice of yoga and meditation, which hones her ability to center herself, breathe, and relax even under high levels of stress and pain.

Making a Successful Commitment to Self-Care

People enroll in the Headache Reduction Program with the goal of learning self-care techniques that build resilience to stress and help control chronic headaches. The support of significant others is an important element in achieving success with this program. Discuss your decision to learn the HARP relaxation and stress reduction techniques with your health-care professionals, family, and friends.

Give yourself time to learn and practice the HARP techniques. Be patient with yourself. Remember that the goal is not to achieve mastery; the goal of relaxation is essentially to let go of demands and expectations for a time each day. *Enjoy your practice.* It provides you with a way to temporarily put aside the burdens and pressures of life in order to restore your inner strength and regain the balance and vitality you need to carry on.

To summarize, success in this program involves the following steps:

Step 1: Understand the migraine disorder and your enhanced responsiveness to stress, as presented in Part I of this book.

Step 2: Recognize the dangers of chronic stress, become aware of your physical and mental stress response, and understand your body's need for daily relaxation periods in order to balance your nervous system and restore resilience to stress and to headaches.

Step 3: Make a commitment to self-care, to learning relaxation techniques, and to integrating them into your daily life.

Step 4: Reach out for support and guidance. Let your family, friends, coworkers, and health-care professionals know that you are involved in a self-care program that complements medical treatment of migraine. You may also wish to become part of a headache support group, by contacting the National Headache Foundation or the American Council for Headache Education.

Step 5: Be patient and compassionate with yourself. "He who is fretted by his own failings will not correct them. All profitable correction comes from a calm, peaceful mind" (Saint Francis de Sales). Trying to relax is like trying to fall asleep: you accomplish your goal when you learn to let go of striving.

7

Taking Control When Migraines Threaten

Watching Out for the Prodrome

A migraine is not a headache that strikes like a bolt of lightning out of the blue. Most people get symptoms that warn them when a headache is approaching, and this period (the prodrome) may begin up to forty-eight hours before the headache begins.

You can use the prodrome—the warning phase of the migraine—to your advantage. By taking precautions in advance of the headache, you can weaken and sometimes even abort head pain. This chapter will teach you how to recognize when you're in the prodromal phase of the headache, and give you a prescription of steps to take to lessen your migraine's impact. You will learn to recognize the early signs of the migraine, and use mindful awareness of your breath, body tension, and mood to manage your headache and take control.

Sensing the Approaching Headache: Storm Warnings Are in Effect

Just as you know that rain is imminent when you see the dark clouds accumulating and smell the ozone in the air, you can also sense changes in your state of being that regularly occur before the head pain hits. These physical and mental signs may include food cravings, irritability, yawning, fatigue, and difficulty concentrating. This phase of migraine is the prodrome. It is helpful to recognize the prodrome as a signal to slow down and take precautionary measures to protect yourself from the headache that's brewing. What symptoms do you experience before a headache's onset? Check off your common warning signals.

Storm Warnings: The Headache Prodrome

The following is a list of prodromal symptoms of migraine that can occur twenty-four to forty-eight hours before a headache strikes. Which symptoms do you have?

_____ **Food cravings (carbohydrates, chocolate, sweets)**

_____ **Irritability, moodiness**

_____ **Stress response: cold hands, tense muscles, shallow breathing**

_____ **Yawning**

_____ **Fatigue**

_____ **Difficulty concentrating**

_____ **Other (fill in personal warning signs):** _____

_____

If you are among the 20 percent of migraine sufferers who experience an aura, you should heed the aura as you would any warning. The aura, like the prodrome, is part of the migraine attack itself. Sometimes the aura comes on abruptly without other warning signs. In this case, we use the aura in the same way as the prodrome to ward off the headache.

Taking Cover—Avoiding Triggers and Counteracting Stress

When a headache threatens, reduce your exposure to known headache triggers and protect yourself from sensory overstimulation. This may include avoiding alcohol and reducing your exposure to bright lights, loud noises, and irritating social situations.

The impending migraine can affect you like any other threat to your well-being. It stimulates your sympathetic nervous system to elicit the stress response: your blood pressure and heart rate increase, your breathing becomes disturbed, your hands become cold, and your thoughts become negative and pessimistic. The muscles of your neck, back, and shoulders tighten, making it even more likely that a painful headache is on the way.

Fortunately, you can learn how to keep the stress response from escalating out of control, and you can break the cycle of stress–tension–headache pain. The Princeton Headache Clinic program provides you with simple techniques and self-care exercises that will enable you to take charge of your body's stress response. Through mindful focus on your breath, your body, and your mind, you can learn to let go of constricted breathing, muscle tension, and negative thoughts.

HARP Technique 1: Letting Go of Constricted Breathing

Most of the time you breathe without conscious control, and your respiratory rhythm reflects your state of mind, activity, and tension level. Your breathing becomes constricted and inhibited when you're stressed out or in pain. Do this little experiment. Make a fist to a count of 1 . . . 2 . . . 3 . . . 4 . . . 5. Tighten that fist as hard as you can. Clench it harder! Now let go. What happens when you tighten your fist? You automatically hold your breath. This is an involuntary response to the challenge or stress—even a minor stress such as tightening your grip. Now begin to pay attention to your breathing pattern when you feel the onset of a headache. Observe the movement of your chest and abdomen. Are you breathing shallowly, high in the chest? Or are you breathing deeply and smoothly, allowing the belly to rise and fall?

Attention to the breath is the basis of all relaxation practice and is essential to full health and well-being. Just by tuning in to your breathing rhythm and allowing your respirations to deepen and your abdomen to soften, you can calm your overcharged nervous system and let go of physical tension, discomfort, and head pain.

HARP Self-Care Exercise: Diaphragmatic Breathing

Practice breath awareness and deep diaphragmatic breathing twice daily when you are headache-free. Here is an exercise that will help you get in tune with your breathing. It works best if you record these instructions for yourself, or ask someone to read them to you in a slow, soothing voice. Daily practice will make deep, full breathing an automatic response when your body senses a headache approaching.

> Start by getting into a comfortable position, either sitting or lying down on your back. Let your body relax and let go of tension, allowing the chair or floor to support your body for now. Allow your eyes to close gently. Then begin to pay attention to your breathing, without trying to change it in any way. Simply observe the breath, tuning in to the rhythm and sensation of breathing. Feel the air as it flows in through your nose and back out again. Feel the temperature of the air you breathe. Listen to the soft sound of the inhalation and the exhalation. Focus on the movement your body makes as it breathes, as air fills the lungs, then is released. Feel the movement of your belly, mid-abdomen, and chest. Now put your hand on your belly as you continue to breathe, and observe its

movement. Try taking a deep breath in through your nose, and let it out through your mouth with a big sigh. Now, breathing in and out through your nose, gently focus on your belly's rise and fall. As you inhale, your belly gently expands as the diaphragm, an internal respiratory muscle, allows deep expansion of the lower lungs. As you breathe, soften your belly. Allow the air to flow in and out freely, without holding back. If you become distracted or find your thoughts wandering away from your focus, simply observe that and passively bring your attention back to the next breath. It feels good to breathe this way, calm and peaceful. The air we breathe enriches the blood with oxygen for every cell; it normalizes the heart rate and balances the blood pressure. Enjoy the feeling of relaxation as you breathe and focus on the rhythm and sensation of your breath.

RX #1: Breath Focus during a Headache

Pain triggers the fight-or-flight response—you tense up and this disturbs your normal breathing. You may hold your breath, or breathe shallowly and fitfully, rather than deeply, smoothly, with a regular rhythm. Diaphragmatic breathing draws air into the lower part of the lungs. This form of breathing is in contrast to shallow breathing in the upper portion of the lungs, the usual response to stress.

To regain control of your breathing during a headache:

Start with a deep, full, stress-relieving breath. Breathe in deeply through your nose, and then let it out through your mouth with a big sigh of relief, saying "Aaaaahhhhhhhhhh." Now breathe in and out through your nose, mindfully following each breath, feeling the temperature of the breath, hearing its sound, being with each breath in and each breath out. To enhance your focus, count down from 4 to 1, saying each number to yourself with each exhalation. If you become distracted, passively return your focus to the sensation of breathing and to counting. Allow yourself to become calmer and more relaxed with each exhalation.

Breathing fully and deeply and consciously helps counteract the stress response. Breath focus is the first step in taking care of yourself and will enable you to take the next steps necessary to regain balance—letting go of the tension in your body and in your mind.

HARP Technique 2: Letting Go of Your Body's Tension

You respond to stress and pain by protectively armoring yourself. Your physical posture becomes defensive; your muscles tense up and prepare for fight or flight. The hassles of daily life and old traumas are carried within your muscles and manifested in constricted posture and facial expressions, like hunched-up shoulders or a clenched jaw. People are often totally unaware of the unnecessary tension they hold in their muscles. Stop for a moment, lift your shoulders up to your ears, and let them drop. Repeat this movement, breathing in as you raise your shoulders up toward your ears, exhaling as you let them drop. Do your shoulders feel a bit lower and looser than they did before?

Learning to relax the body is important in both preventing and relieving headache pain. Stress-induced muscle tension, particularly in the neck, shoulders, scalp, and jaw, is a common headache trigger. After the head pain starts, the body automatically tenses up even more. This response increases discomfort and pain, which leads to persistent body tension, a vicious cycle. Learning body focus and relaxation skills can help you break through the stress–tension–headache cycle.

HARP Self-Care Exercise: Body Scan

The body scan is a systematic method of tuning in to the body. While breathing and focusing on each area of the body, pay attention to the sensations and feelings in each part. As you breathe in and out, allow the energy of your breath to circulate freely, energizing, warming, and releasing tension in every muscle.

This exercise should be practiced daily when headache free. You will experience how your body feels when completely relaxed, so you can return to that state quickly when stressed by a headache. You may wish to read this guided meditation into a tape recorder, or have someone read it to you in a calm, slow, and soothing manner.

Sit or lie down in a comfortable position. Allow your eyelids to drop. Start with a deep breath, exhaling with a sigh. Then passively pay attention to your breathing, coming in through your nostrils, and going out. Allow your breathing to become full and naturally deepen.

Inhale deeply and slowly, bringing the breath up into your head. With each exhalation let go of muscle tension in your scalp . . . your forehead . . . your brow . . . the muscles around your eyes . . . your mouth and jaw. Take as many breaths as you need to gently release all the stress that has gathered in these areas.

Now focus your attention to your neck, shoulders, and back, bringing the breath into these areas fully and completely. As you exhale, feel your muscles soften, becoming warm and heavy. With each breath, the muscles in the neck, shoulders, and back are becoming warmer and more relaxed.

Inhale, and bring the breath into your arms, down into your hands and fingers. Let any tension leave with each exhalation. Continue to breathe slowly and deeply. Enjoy the feeling of warmth and relaxation in your arms, hands, and fingers.

Focus on your chest, abdomen, and pelvis. Breathe into these areas, loosening and softening any muscle tension, allowing relaxed, free movement as you breathe in and out. You're nourishing and nurturing your body by breathing quietly and deeply. Your respirations allow life-giving oxygen to surge through your bloodstream, and with every exhalation your body releases unnecessary toxins and tension. You are restoring your body and bringing a pink, healthy glow to every organ, including your skin.

Now focus on your legs and feet. Carry the breath in and direct it down toward your legs, paying attention to the sensations you feel. With each exhalation, allow all tension to dissolve. Your legs feel heavy and warm. You feel renewed circulation and warmth in your feet and toes.

Enjoy the feeling of relaxation throughout your body. Your body feels refreshed, your mind serenely aware. You've given yourself a healthy gift, the restful time you need to restore balance and well-being.

RX #2: Body Focus during a Headache

Pay attention to the way you physically react when you have a headache. Pain causes an automatic increase in muscle tension. Check for tension throughout your body—particularly, tune in to your body's sensations. What do you feel? Openly and gently, yield to your pain. Trying to deny, fight, or ignore pain serves no purpose but to perpetuate it. When you know it's a migraine, and you have the sense that it's going to be a bad one, take your pain medication early on—don't wait for it to be unbearable. Your medication will work faster and more effectively when taken at the onset of the headache. The best results occur when you take the following self-care action as well:

To release body tension during a headache, use your breath. Sit or lay down in a quiet place, and give yourself a few minutes to let go of your pain. Breathe in to the area that's tense and uncomfortable, and allow the tension to flow out with each exhalation. As you breathe in, visualize the breath moving right up to your head and scalp, bringing soothing, cooling oxygen to the rescue. Soften the muscles in your abdomen, chest, and shoulders, so you can breathe deeply and fully. Continue breathing to the tense areas until you feel your head relaxing, softening, gently letting go of tension and pain. Then visualize your breath bringing healing oxygen to your face . . . your jaw . . . your neck . . . your shoulders . . . arms . . . hands . . . back . . . belly . . . and legs. Focus on breathing in healing, rejuvenating, soothing oxygen to those tense places, and breathing out the tension and pain. With each breath, you will become more relaxed. You will loosen the tethers of pain and tension, and recover from your migraine more quickly.

HARP Technique 3: Letting Go of Negative Thoughts

What goes through your mind when you have a headache? You may think, "Oh no! I can't be getting a headache now. I have an important day ahead, and I can't miss work. My coworkers (or family, or friends) are going to kill me; they can never depend on me. I hate these headaches! What did I do wrong to bring this one on? I should know better than to have two beers with dinner and go to bed late. Should I give in and take pain medication? I'm afraid of all the side effects. I can't make any plans without these migraines coming around to spoil everything."

Do you hear the emotional content behind these statements? They reflect feelings of disappointment, anger, self-blame, guilt, pessimism, and despair. In a study published in the medical journal *Headache*, fifty migraine sufferers were asked to recall their thoughts and emotions during their last migraine headache. Forty-one of the patients described negative feelings and thoughts during a migraine attack, and many said that their emotional state of mind was as intense as the head pain itself.

Negative thinking is part of the stress response. Thinking that the absolute worst will happen may be protective when we're preparing for fighting off or fleeing from an enemy. But when the threat to our well-being is a headache, negative thoughts make a bad situation worse.

RX #3: Mind Focus during a Headache

Fortunately, once you become aware that negative thoughts occur automatically when you're enduring stress or pain, you can look at these thoughts objectively and choose to let go of their grip. One way to do this is to identify the cognitive distortions in these automatic thoughts and counter them with more constructive self-talk. This is a technique known as cognitive therapy, and it has been developed as a drug-free treatment for depression and many other psychological problems.

Here's how to apply cognitive repair to the damaging negative headache thoughts described above:

"My coworkers/family/friends are going to kill me, they can never depend on me."

Ask yourself, "Is that true?" Watch out for absolute words like "never" and the tendency to exaggerate or catastrophize. Another common distortion is to mind-read or predict that others won't be understanding or forgiving. Would *you* be that unsupportive and insensitive if a coworker were in the same situation? Often we are much harder on ourselves than we are on others.

Self-healing thought:

The people in my life understand that I have migraines. Right now I need to take care of myself to get over this headache, and then I'll be back on track.

"What did I do wrong? I should never have . . ."

Being self-critical during a headache is like blaming the victim or kicking a person when he or she is already down. Headaches are not completely under one's control. We can learn to avoid some triggers, but there are many factors—like weather changes or hormonal fluctuations—that are independent of our control. If you've done something you know triggers headaches, give yourself a break. Sometimes a small or occasional lapse (for example, a half glass of wine on weekends) can be tolerated without getting a headache. When things don't work out, and you're suffering from a headache, don't blame yourself for being human. You deserve compassion. Let it start with your own self-talk.

Self-healing thought:

Now is not the time to blame; blame is negative and nonproductive. Right now I need to let go of self-blame and focus on self-healing.

"Should I give in and take my pain medication? I'm afraid of side effects."

It's common for migraine sufferers to have negative or ambivalent feelings about taking drugs. People often wait until the pain has reached the point that it is disabling. They take a drug not so much to relieve the pain as to be able to carry on. Often when the headache first starts, they convince themselves that this isn't a migraine, it's "just tension" or "sinuses." Yet, the majority of time, migraine sufferers know early on when it's a migraine headache—especially if they also recognize a familiar pattern or trigger (like right before menstruation, after a skipped meal, or when there's been a change in atmospheric pressure). You should respect your migraine "instinct" and take immediate self-care action. Give yourself a break from needless suffering and treat your migraine as early as possible.

Medications taken at the onset of a headache work more effectively. Think of your headache as a cascading process; if you interrupt it at the start, it is easier to gain control of the pain. If you have any questions about drug side effects, talk with your health-care practitioner or pharmacist. Taking a pain medication when needed is not "giving in"—it's another way to take care of yourself and recover more quickly.

Self-healing thought:

The earlier I take my medication, the better it will work. If I combine the HARP relaxation techniques with medication, I will get the best result.

Should I or Shouldn't I?: More on the Decision to Take Medication

• If you're taking pain medications for headaches more than three times a week, analgesic rebound can occur. Breaking the cycle of rebound headaches is often difficult to accomplish without medical help. If you are worried that you are taking pain medications too frequently, keep a headache diary and consult your health-care practitioner or a headache specialist. You may need the additional support of preventive medications to decrease headache frequency.

• Don't confuse your fear of a headache with the actual signals of a developing headache. The fear and anticipation of a headache can lead to taking analgesics to "prevent" a headache from occurring. This is an inappropriate use of medication and can result in overuse of over-the-counter or prescription drugs.

• If your migraines are severe but infrequent, early judicious use of a painkiller or a triptan drug, coupled with HARP relaxation techniques, is the most effective response.

• If you usually get a severe headache following an aura, early use of medication together with HARP relaxation techniques is the most appropriate step. The aura may trigger a stress response, due to the unsettling experience of having visual or other perceptual distortions and the anticipation of the headache to follow. Relaxation methods will counteract this developing stress response.

The Role of Sleep in Pain Relief

Sleep is the natural way the brain has of terminating a migraine attack. The response to sleep is most vividly seen in children. Distressed, in pain, and nauseated from a migraine, a child may fall asleep for an hour or two. On awaking, the headache is gone and the child's first question may be "What's for dinner, Mom?" The restoration by sleep is in sync with the concept that the headache forces you to rest and withdraw. This rapid response of the migraine to sleep, however, becomes less vigorous with age.

After the Headache Storm: the Postdrome

You have now seen how a migraine has several phases, the prodrome, the aura (in the 10 to 20 percent of migraineurs who get auras), and then the headache. After the headache terminates, many people experience a final phase, the postdrome. In this stage, the worst of the head pain is over, but many people experience an aftereffect. They describe it like a "headache shadow," the "headache remains," or a "hangover." Some people experience a sense of elation, a "high" from the remaining endorphins (the body's natural painkillers). It is important to remain vigilant and take extra self-care precautions for twenty-four hours after the headache subsides. Your migraine threshold is still low, which can render you at greater risk for another storm to hit.

When your headache is over, continue to avoid triggers and reduce unnecessary stimulation. Pass up that glass of wine or excuse yourself from an optional social engagement. Use brief periods of diaphragmatic breathing if you feel the headache coming back. Gently stretch any areas of the body that remain tender or in spasm, such as the neck and shoulders. In the headache's aftermath, accept the need to rest and recover. Without self-judgment or blame, see if this headache gave you any clues as to what its triggers were. Remember, headache triggers are usually a mix of things you can't control (like hormonal or weather changes) with things you can control (like diet or hours of sleep). Ask yourself: Am I getting regular sleep, exercise, meals? Am I taking time to practice relaxation daily? Learning from your headaches and making necessary lifestyle changes will make you healthier, protect your nervous system, and render you more headache resilient.

Summary of HARP Techniques

• Know your headache warning signals and take action early on, before the headache gets bad. Protect yourself by avoiding triggers—loud sounds, bright lights, alcohol, or skipped meals.

• Take your pain medication early if you know this is a migraine, but don't substitute medication for the HARP techniques. These self-care exercises enhance pain relief dramatically, by helping you let go of constricted breathing, muscle tension, and negative thoughts.

• RX #1—Breath Focus: Start with a deep breath in through your nose, and exhale out through your mouth with a big sigh of relief—ahhhhhh. Then continue focused breathing in and out through your nose, counting backward from 4 to 1.

• RX #2—Body Focus: Sit or lie down in a comfortable place, and take a few minutes to tune in to the tension in your body. Breathe in and visualize bringing healing oxygen to the tense areas in your head, scalp, face, jaw, neck, shoulders, back, arms, and legs. Exhale fully and deeply, releasing pain and tension with each breath out.

• RX #3—Mind Focus: Stress and pain automatically skew your mind to think pessimistically, adding insult to injury. Shake off these thoughts once you recognize that they are unproductive and counter them with supportive, self-healing thoughts. Say to yourself: I accept the fact that I have migraines, and other people understand this, too. Right now, I need to focus on taking care of myself, so I can get over this headache just as I have done before.

8

Natural Ways to Prevent Headaches

The art of migraine prevention is to identify and avoid specific headache triggers while at the same time raising the threshold for getting a migraine. You can do this by protecting your sensitive nervous system from sensory overload and excessive tension—and still have a life!

One emerging theory of migraine is that the headache is the brain's way of protecting itself from overload. Migraine pain is often disabling—the sufferer has no choice but to rest and withdraw. Fortunately, you can use techniques of self-care to prevent the excessive buildup of charge and tension in the nervous system and still maintain your vitality. The HARP techniques all involve different ways of inducing the Relaxation Response—the antidote to stress and anxiety. By counterbalancing stress with periods of relaxation, you can raise the threshold for triggering a headache and become headache resilient.

This chapter outlines a program of self-care to prevent migraines including:

- Paying attention to regular daily routines including sleep, meals, and exercise.

- Avoiding sensory overload that can "trip" the migraine switch, and heeding the warning signs when you are particularly "migraine vulnerable."
- Identifying specific migraine triggers with the help of a headache diary, and then doing what you can to avoid triggering substances or situations.
- Making relaxation breaks a "health habit," by learning how to integrate HARP techniques—such as diaphragmatic breathing, meditation, mindfulness, the body scan, and yoga—into even the busiest lifestyle.

Identifying Headache Triggers

Because your nervous system is more responsive and more easily stimulated than the nervous system of someone without migraines, you are more sensitive to change than average. Stress occurs whenever we are forced to adapt to change. Weekend headaches reflect such sensitivity to change—in this case a change in stress level from a busy week to a relaxing weekend.

All nature functions in cycles of activity—the day-night cycle and the yearly seasons are all predictable cycles. You can think of your daily "routine" as such a cycle. There is a predictability to it, and the body becomes conditioned to respond to regular cycles of activity. In this way, you adapt to a routine of sleeping, working, eating, and recreation. Predictability lessens stress as your response becomes automatic. Deviation (particularly sudden change) from the routine of daily activity can be stressful and trigger headache. That's why so many headache sufferers complain of headaches during the first few days of vacation; they are adjusting to a new schedule of sleep, meals, and activities.

Of course, life is not always predictable and you do not always have control over all of your stressors. Factors outside your control that can trigger headaches include changes in weather, environmental and atmospheric changes, world events, and internal changes such as the hormonal fluctuations that are part of the normal menstrual cycle in women.

This doesn't mean that because you have migraines, you are forced to lead a dull and colorless existence so as not to get headaches. A balanced approach offers a middle path to preventing headaches. This involves identifying and controlling some of the factors that trigger headaches while at the same time raising one's headache threshold with the regular use of relaxation exercises.

Using a Headache Diary

Headache specialists often request that their patients keep a diary or headache log. This serves several purposes, by providing

1. A record of the number of headaches. People often suppress memory of pain, so it is difficult to recall how many headaches occurred last month. Also, most migraine sufferers will remember only their severe headaches. A headache log records all headache types and indicates how active the headaches really are.

2. A record of painkiller use. This is particularly helpful to the health-care practitioner in determining the most effective headache relief and identifying excessive dependency on painkillers or analgesic rebound syndrome.

3. The impact of headaches on your quality of life. You can record the times that headaches limited your ability to work or interfered with social plans.

4. An aid in pattern recognition and identifying headache triggers.

To provide this information, a headache log should contain:

- A record of each headache
- A record of head pain severity. A "0–3" scale is useful with

zero indicating no headache, 1=mild, 2=moderate, and 3=severe. For children we often simplify this by using a capital "H" for a bad headache and a lowercase "h" for a milder headache. This also works well for adults.

- An indication of the duration of the headache in hours, and the time that the headache began (for example, arising out of sleep, upon waking, or later in the day)
- What relief measures were taken (rest, ice packs, medication, relaxation techniques)
- The factors that may have triggered this headache (such as a skipped meal, a glass of wine, or a late night out)
- In women, a notation of the menstrual cycle

The simpler the log is, the better. This information can be recorded on a kitchen calendar, in a diary, in a notebook, or on a computer.

Here are some of the more commonly recognized patterns identified by headache logs:

- Weekend headaches
- Headaches occurring only at times of stress, or following stress
- Headaches arising from sleep (if this is a change in headache pattern, notify your health-care practitioner)
- Menstrual migraines
- Frequent tension-type headaches occurring between migraines (this may indicate a transforming migraine pattern)
- Frequent use of painkillers in anticipation of headache (this often indicates an emerging or potential analgesic rebound situation)
- Headaches triggered by certain dietary or other agents

Once the pattern is recognized, more specific steps can be taken to reduce the known triggers—whether it is stress, sensory overload, irregular sleep, painkiller use, alcohol, or certain foods.

Watching Out for Sensory Overload

When you are exposed to repeated stimulation of bright lights or loud sounds, your brain normally responds by becoming less sensitive to the repeated stimulus. Many migraine sufferers are unable to filter out or habituate to repetitive stimulation. When your nervous system is excessively stimulated or overloaded, a migraine may result, which forces you to withdraw from the stimulus and to shut down.

This increased sensitivity to stimulus accounts for why bright lights, loud sounds, and strong smells such as solvents, perfumes, and cigarette smoke can trigger a migraine.

Here are some ways to avoid overstimulation:

- Limit your exposure to bright flickering lights such as fluorescent lighting.
- Use a filter on your computer screen.
- Wear ear plugs at the next rock concert you attend.
- Wear sunglasses on bright days.
- Limit time in situations that are stressful, such as crowded malls.
- Avoid watching television late at night, as brain excitation interferes with natural relaxation.

Food Triggers

Food and dietary triggers for migraine are often overemphasized. Recent studies suggest that less than 25 percent of migraine episodes are triggered by food or alcohol. The reaction to certain foods is unique to the individual and is usually not an allergy or immune mechanism. Most food or alcohol triggers will induce a headache within twenty-four hours of exposure and are identifiable on a headache log.

The following is a list of some foods that are commonly

associated with triggering migraine. This list is useful as a reference. We do not advise a restrictive or "headache diet" but rather a rational avoidance of foods that you have found to trigger your headaches.

Remember, the shifting headache threshold may account for why a headache can be triggered by a certain food at one time, but not every time.

Common Food Triggers

Aged cheese
Monosodium glutamate (MSG)
Processed fish and meats or those containing nitrates, such as
    hot dogs
Dark chocolate
Aspartame (artificial sweetener)
Certain alcoholic beverages (particularly red wine)
Citrus fruits
Caffeine

The craving for certain foods, as part of the migraine prodrome, sometimes complicates trying to identify food triggers. This is particularly the case with carbohydrate craving. The sudden desire to eat chocolate may be part of the developing migraine, and not a food trigger.

Four Basic Rules for Avoiding a Headache

1. *Stick to a regular sleep routine.* A change in sleep patterns is often a headache trigger. Sleep deprivation increases stress levels, rendering you more headache vulnerable. On the other hand,

oversleeping—an extra hour or two in the morning—is enough to bring on a headache as well. This is one of the causes of the "weekend headache." It is often worth sacrificing that extra hour or two of sleep to maintain a regular sleep pattern and prevent a headache.

Optimal sleep requirements vary with age and with the individual. You probably know how much sleep you need to function effectively and should try to stay as close to that requirement as possible. And remember to practice your relaxation techniques every night: they are the drug-free cure for insomnia.

2. *Don't skip meals.* The triggering of a migraine by skipping meals is often misdiagnosed as low blood sugar or hypoglycemia. In reality, skipping meals is itself a stressor that will trigger a headache in susceptible migraine sufferers. Under time pressure during the busy workweek, many people sacrifice their routine. A common example is skipping breakfast when running late for work. Again, simple attention to routine can reduce a headache trigger.

3. *Get off the couch.* Regular exercise can prevent headaches by making you more headache resistant. The exercise can be as simple as taking a fifteen- or twenty-minute walk four times a week. Vigorous exercise, such as running, swimming, or working out at a gym, is also beneficial. Stress and time pressure are the most common reasons for not exercising regularly—just when it is needed most. Exercise is even more effective as a headache preventive when it is something you look forward to and enjoy.

4. *Let go of stress; let go of headaches.* At the Princeton Headache Clinic, we have found that people need to learn how to relax, and this doesn't mean just mastering techniques. It also means acquiring a new state of mind, a change in perception. Don't view relaxation as self-indulgent, or "doing nothing." Taking time out to relax and refresh your nervous system is a daily necessity for self-preservation—for headache control, enhanced health, and well-being.

Headache Reduction through Relaxation

Relaxation methods help to prevent migraine even if the headache is not triggered by stress. Relaxation produces a physiological change in the body and raises the headache threshold. Regular relaxation is analogous to the use of medication to prevent migraine, but without side effects.

You certainly can't get rid of all of life's daily annoyances and responsibilities, but you can learn how to give yourself relaxation breaks—periods of time in which you can let go of worries and tension. Herbert Benson, M.D., the cardiologist and founder of the Mind/Body Medical Institute in Boston, has spent over twenty-five years studying the body's antidote to stress, the Relaxation Response. Dr. Benson found that just twenty minutes of relaxation per day had profound health benefits, including lowering blood pressure, maintaining immunity, and promoting sleep.

You may be thinking, "Twenty minutes—no way can I find that kind of time." Like learning any new skill, it takes effort at first, as you consciously have to remind yourself to take the time for a relaxation break. After a while, you can take these breaks without even thinking about it. Just as it has become automatic to brush your teeth before bedtime to prevent tooth decay, you will find yourself focusing on diaphragmatic breathing whenever you are in a tense situation. And relaxation breaks are self-rewarding. They make you feel better immediately. As you become more tuned in to states of tension in your body, you will seek the relief and well-being these breaks give you. You will find that if you don't take time for yourself, you will spend even more time feeling tense and miserable.

Start with Your Favorite Diversions
Many of our patients find that they are already taking relaxation breaks, without recognizing them as such. Whenever you focus

on one thing at a time, and free your mind of distracting thoughts, you are eliciting the Relaxation Response. Liz takes a relaxation break whenever she walks her dog; she tunes in to the antics of her pet, the way he stops and sniffs and enjoys the air blowing through the leaves. When Ian goes to the gym after work and gets on the treadmill, he takes a relaxation break when he focuses on the repetitive movement of his strides, his rhythmic breathing in and out, and the warm sensation in his muscles as he exercises. David takes time during his daily train commute for a stress break; he sits back, closes his eyes, and focuses on the repetitive motion of the train, the in and out of his breathing, while loosening up muscle tension and breathing freely.

There are just two requirements to elicit relaxation—first, a focus of attention on a word, breath, or activity that is repetitive and absorbing, and second, a mindful return to that focus when the brain's unceasing thoughts jump around to other things. Think about what you enjoy focusing on and find soothing, whether it's needlework, swimming, or playing a drum. The next time you do these activities, make sure they become valued periods of time when you free yourself from any distractions or any worrisome thoughts.

Even Short Breaks Do the Job

There are two types of relaxation breaks: short "minute" breaks you can take in the midst of a busy day, and extended breaks you take for longer periods (ten to twenty minutes) once or twice a day. The short breaks keep the stresses of the day from building up. They give you a quick way to deal with stress so your nervous system can return to normal—ready and able to face the next stressor. Extended breaks give you the opportunity to relax more deeply. These breaks act as a point of reference or touchstone, a state of total relaxation the body remembers and can quickly return to when necessary. Relaxation breaks are healthy for you in three ways: they balance the overwrought nervous system, build resilience to headaches, and restore your sense of optimism and well-being.

HARP Techniques for Headache Prevention

Focus #1: Mindful Breathing and Meditation

Meditation is the practice of focused awareness for a sustained period. It has been employed as a healing practice since ancient times. The subjects of Dr. Herbert Benson's early research on relaxation were practitioners of transcendental meditation. Meditation uses the breath as an anchor of attention, often coupled with counting the breaths, or repeating a mantra—a special word, phrase, or prayer.

Practicing Breath Focus Techniques
A drop of experience is worth a gallon of theory—in other words, the best way to learn meditation is by practicing it.

Here are three ways to meditate:

1. *Breath awareness.* Focus on the physical sensation of breathing. Get comfortable. Sit or lie down and adjust your body until you can just let go into the chair or mat. Then take a deep breath in, hold it for two to three seconds, and then let it go completely. Try breathing in through your nose and out through your mouth. Take a big sigh of relief. Then continue breathing in and out through your nostrils, and focus on "being with" the breath as you inhale and as you exhale, hearing its quiet flow, feeling its warmth. Relax all of your muscles, loosen your belly, and yield to the flow of air moving in and out. Start by meditating for approximately five minutes. Don't set a timer or have a clock ticking away beside you. Build up to ten minutes once or twice daily, then up to twenty minutes once or twice per day.

2. *Meditate with a mantra.* Next, try focused breathing along with repeating a word or phrase. A mantra is like a broom that "sweeps away" distracting thoughts. Simply say to yourself "breathing in" as you inhale, "breathing out" as you exhale. You can also try using words that give a sense of peace and unity with nature such as "blue sky," "cool mountain," "quiet canyon." Words that invoke a spiritual belief or consciousness, like "Hail Mary," "Peace," "Let it be," "Shalom," or the Sanskrit words "hom-sah," meaning "I am that," are especially powerful when given the added dimension of belief.

3. *Counting with the breath.* Inhale silently, counting slowly to 4, hold your breath a couple seconds, then exhale fully, counting backward from 4 to 1. Pause, then repeat. Note that the breath has four parts: inhale, pause, exhale, pause. These pauses are the still, quiet times of the breath. Allow yourself to be still, and enjoy the peacefulness of these moments.

With practice, the relaxation response becomes easier and easier to produce. You can use your favorite technique for taking short "minute" breaks throughout the day.

Focus #2: Moving Mindfully
Western culture tends to make people top-heavy. Your focus is caught up "in your head," preoccupied with worries about what you have to do next. You walk from your car to the grocery store without any notice of the contact your feet make with the pavement. The demands of daily living cause you to lose touch with your body's sensations and needs.

The Eastern world has given us the antidote to stress, through the time-tested healing practices of tai chi, yoga, and qigong. These ancient philosophies provide exercises that are designed to release and mobilize body energy that is stuck or dammed up. The flowing way you move and breathe will help you relax and bring your mind's focus into the present moment.

Practicing Body Focus Techniques

1. Try this qigong exercise, which balances the agitated nervous system by moving the energy down out of your head and into your body's center.

> Standing with arms at your sides, begin by lifting your arms with palms up over your head, inhaling deeply and imagining that your hands are scooping or gathering the surrounding energy in the atmosphere. Once your arms are all the way up overhead, bring your fingertips together and allow your hands to drift down slowly, smoothing out your body's agitated energy field, finally placing your hands gently on your belly. Now breathe into your center, softening and allowing your belly to expand as you inhale and deflate as you exhale, for four deep mindful breaths.

2. Any rhythmic movement with awareness can induce relaxation. Walking, jogging, or swimming performed with awareness and pleasure will counteract stress. As you move, count each step or stroke to a 1 . . . 2 . . . 3 . . . 4 rhythm or count your breath repeatedly as you move. The focus of awareness on the movement places the mind and body in unison and induces a state of relaxation. The feeling of pleasure is a sure sign that you are beginning to relax.

3. The body scan is a systematic method of tuning in to the body. While breathing and focusing on each area of the body, you bring attention to the sensations and feelings in each part. Allow the energy of the breath to circulate freely, energizing, warming, and releasing tension in the muscles.

> Sit or lie down in a comfortable position. Allow your eyelids to drop. Start with a deep breath, exhaling with a sigh. Then passively pay attention to your breathing, coming in through your nostrils, and going out again—effortlessly, like gentle ocean waves against the sandy shore. Allow your breathing to become full and naturally deepen.

Inhale deeply and slowly, bringing the breath up into your head. With each exhalation let go of muscle tension in your scalp . . . your forehead . . . your brow . . . the muscles around your eyes . . . your mouth and jaw. Take as many breaths as you need to gently release all the stress that has gathered in these areas. Now focus your attention on your neck, shoulders, and back, bringing the breath into these areas fully and completely. As you exhale, feel your muscles soften, becoming warm and heavy. With each breath, the muscles in your neck, shoulders, and back are becoming warmer and more relaxed.

Inhale, and bring the air into your arms, down into your hands and fingers. Let any tension leave with each exhalation. Continue to breathe slowly and deeply. Enjoy the feeling of warmth and relaxation in your arms, hands, and fingers.

Focus on your chest, abdomen, and pelvis. Breathe into these areas, loosening and softening any muscle tension, allowing relaxed, free movement as you breathe in and out. You are nourishing and nurturing your body by breathing quietly and deeply. Your respirations allow life-giving oxygen to surge through your bloodstream, and with every exhalation your body releases unnecessary toxins and tension. You are restoring your body and bringing a pink, healthy glow to every cell, tissue, and organ.

Now focus on your legs and feet. Carry the breath in and direct it down toward your legs, paying attention to the sensations you feel. With each exhalation, allow all tension to dissolve—your legs feel heavy and warm; you feel renewed circulation and warmth in your feet and toes.

Enjoy the feeling of relaxation throughout your body. Your body feels refreshed; your mind is serenely aware. You've given yourself an essential gift, the restful time you need to restore your balance and your resiliency to stress.

4. Yoga for Headache Reduction: The HARP exercises are drawn from yoga, qigong, and tai chi. Yoga has become part of our popular culture; it's made the cover of popular magazines, and Hollywood stars and television talk show hosts sing its praises. Many of us feel rather intimidated by photos we've seen of the

pretzel-like maneuvers of practicing gurus, yet yoga can be adapted to people of every age group and medical condition. At the Princeton Headache Clinic, we teach yoga exercises that are simple, yet have powerful benefits. Yoga is a systematic way of focusing your mind, body, and breath. It gives you a way to take relaxation breaks that enhance flexibility, balance, strength, and concentration.

The HARP yoga series is divided into three sets of exercises: standing, spinal, and sitting. Take the time to practice yoga for extended breaks, but keep in mind that postures can be used individually for short breaks when you feel tension creeping into your muscles during your busy day.

STANDING SERIES

1. *The upright position:* Stand with your feet flat on the floor, your toes pointing forward. Feel the sensation of the floor beneath your feet. Lift your toes up and down, and notice how the bones and muscles in your feet help balance your body. Your arms are down at your sides; your shoulders feel loose and relaxed. Focus your eyes forward. As you breathe, allow your spine to stretch and "grow" upward toward the ceiling, your head balanced easily at the top of the spine, your chin level with the floor, your jaw and facial muscles relaxed. Enjoy the dignity and grace of standing straight and tall. Remain in this posture while you breathe fully for three to five breaths. (See Fig. 8.1.)

2. *The head nod (Yes!):* Tilt your head forward by slowly moving your chin down toward your chest. Feel the stretch at the back of your neck. Then slowly lift your chin back up, raising it upward about forty-five degrees, and feel the stretch in your neck. Repeat this movement, slowly tilting your head down and up, nodding your head in a big YES. Breathe rhythmically, breathing in as your chin moves up, breathing out as your chin moves down. Do three repetitions. (See Fig. 8.2.)

3. From the standing position, bend forward, and place your

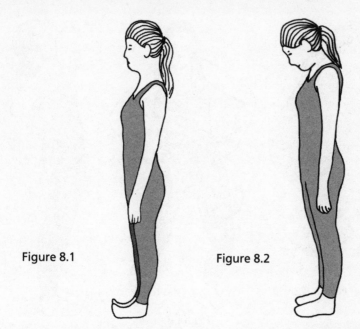

Figure 8.1   Figure 8.2

hands on your knees, with knees bent comfortably. Holding on to your knees, rotate them four times in one direction, then reverse. Focus on the sensation in your feet, ankles, and legs, as you increase their mobility and reduce stiffness. (See Fig. 8.3.)

4. Standing upright, place your hands on your hips. Then rotate your hips Hula Hoop style, four times to the right and four times to the left. Loosen up your waist, hips, and legs, and enjoy the sensation of freeing up tension in the waist, hips, and pelvis. (See Fig. 8.4.)

5. Standing with legs hip-width apart for balance, place your hands on your back, palms at your waist, and fingers down. Lift your chin up, stretch and bend backward, looking up. Hold this stretch and breathe. Feel the expansion in your chest and shoulders. Release the stretch, bringing your arms back to your sides, face forward, and breathe. Repeat this backward stretch again. (See Fig. 8.5.)

6. Start in the standing position and allow your arms to hang in front of you as you bend forward, bending your knees. Bend

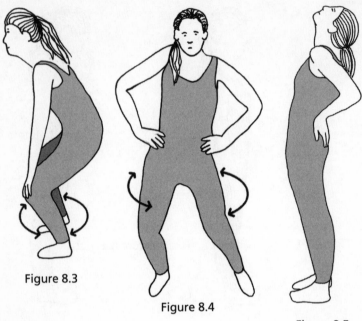

Figure 8.3

Figure 8.4

Figure 8.5

over as far as you can, without strain or pain, and keep your shoulders and arms loose and relaxed. Feel the release of tension in your lower back. Remain in the hanging-down position and breathe two to three breaths. Then very slowly stand upright, feel your back unfolding vertebra by vertebra. Repeat this forward stretch. (See Figs. 8.6a and 8.6b.)

7. Stand up straight, with your feet shoulder-width apart, eyes forward, and arms at your sides. Then twist to the right, looking over your right shoulder, swinging your arms to the right (left arm in front and right arm in back) and then, twisting to the left, look back over your left shoulder, swinging your arms to the left. Breathe and move rhythmically, letting your arms swing loosely, banging against your body like empty shirtsleeves. (See Fig. 8.7.)

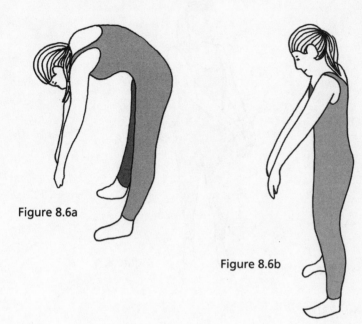

Figure 8.6a

Figure 8.6b

8. Stand. Stretch your arms up overhead. Reach one arm, then the other, and bring them back down to your sides. Lift your arms up overhead as you inhale, then exhale as your arms move down. Repeat three times. End by lifting your arms up again, looking up at your hands while you bring your fingertips together. Then slowly float your hands down to your belly. Place your hands below your navel, and breathe diaphragmatically. Breathe in and out slowly and fully, softening your abdominal muscles, and letting your belly expand as you inhale. Gently contract as you exhale. Continue breathing in and out to that special area below your navel, considered your center of energy, or *dantien*. (See Figs. 8.8a, 8.8b, 8.8c, and 8.8d.)

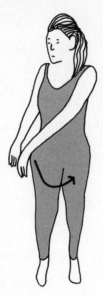

Figure 8.7

SPINAL SERIES

Mobilizing your spine by moving in all directions frees up your body's energy and restores your circulation. Practicing this spinal series can help balance your nervous system, relieve tension in your neck, shoulders, and back, and restore your sense of well-being. Try the following exercises at the end of the day, and feel relaxed and ready for a peaceful night's sleep.

1. Lie down on your back, arms at your sides, palms up. Breathe, and allow yourself to rest completely, letting go of the need to "do something" other than this restorative yoga practice. Feel yourself sinking into the mat; let go of muscle tension, and allow the floor to hold you up. Focus on your breath, breathing fully without constriction; feel your abdomen rise and fall. After three to five deep relaxing breaths, stretch your arms overhead along the floor, stretching your back and lengthening your spine against the floor. Hold this stretch for three seconds, and then

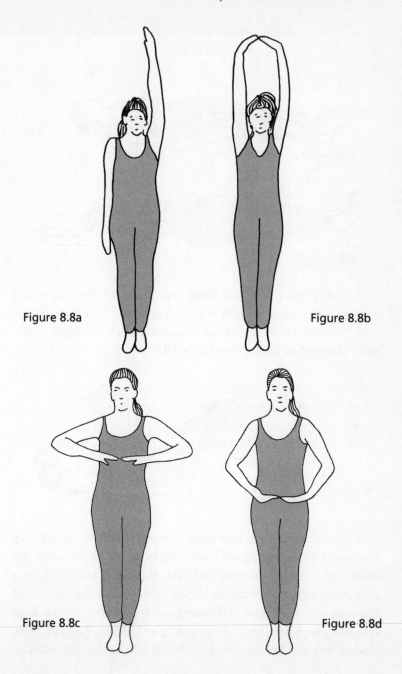

Figure 8.8a

Figure 8.8b

Figure 8.8c

Figure 8.8d

release your muscles, relax, and breathe. Repeat this exercise three times. (See Figs. 8.9a and 8.9b.)

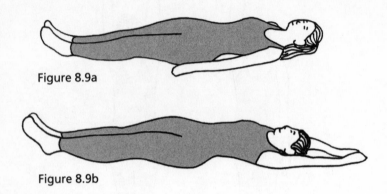

Figure 8.9a

Figure 8.9b

2. Lie on your back and bring your knees up, feet flat on the floor. Breathe out as you tilt your pelvis upward and flatten your back to the floor, and breathe in as you release. Repeat this movement three to six times. (See Fig. 8.10.)

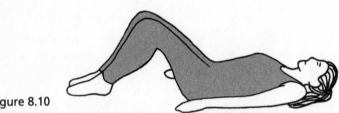

Figure 8.10

3. Lie on your back, then bend your right knee and bring it up to your chest, holding your knee with both hands. Focus on the stretch in your leg muscles and take three full breaths. Lower your right leg to the floor and relax. When you're ready, repeat this exercise with your left knee, and rest. Finally, bring both knees to your chest, your arms circling your knees, hugging them toward you, and breathe for three breaths. While in this position,

rock gently from side to side, loosening up and warming the muscles along your spine. (See Figs. 8.11a and 8.11b.) Release your knees, stretch out your legs, and relax. Feel the release of tension in your back.

Figure 8.11a

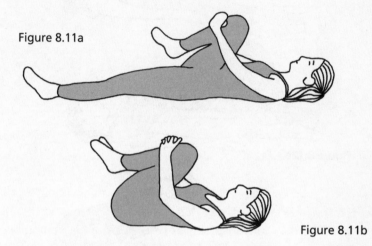

Figure 8.11b

4. Lie on your back with your knees up, feet flat on the floor. Tilt your pelvis, flattening your lower back to the floor, then slowly lift your buttocks up off the floor, bringing your midsection up, forming a diagonal line between your knees and shoulders. Hold this position for three breaths, and then slowly bring your back down to the floor, one vertebra at a time. Repeat three times. (See Figs. 8.12a and 8.12b.)

5. Roll over onto your hands and knees, hands flat on the mat, fingers spread apart and pointing straight ahead. Do the pelvic tilt, also known as the cat, breathing in rhythm with your movement. As you breathe in, your chin moves up, your eyes gaze straight ahead, and your spine curves downward. As you breathe out, tuck your chin down toward your chest, arching your back upward. Repeat this movement three times. (See Figs. 8.13a and 8.13b.)

6. Starting on all fours, with hands lined up under your shoulders, "walk" your hands one step forward, and then lower your

Figure 8.12a

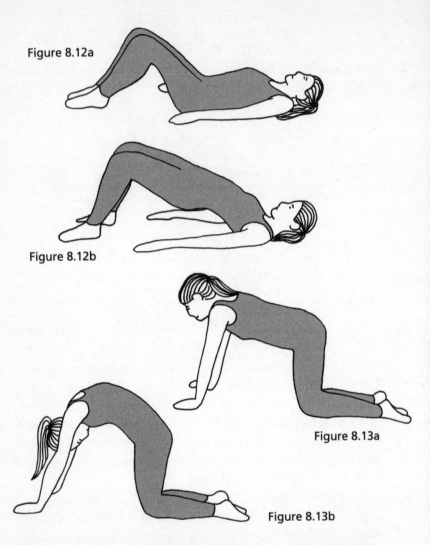

Figure 8.12b

Figure 8.13a

Figure 8.13b

chest down to the floor (like a modified push-up). From this prone position, with your hands on either side of your chest, lift your chin up, arching backward, and move into the "cobra" pose. Then slide your elbows forward to support yourself in the "sphinx" pose. Your eyes gazing straight ahead, breathe for three to five breaths. (See Figs. 8.14a, 8.14b, and 8.14c.)

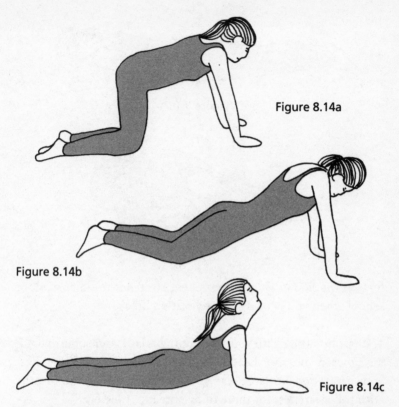

Figure 8.14a

Figure 8.14b

Figure 8.14c

7. Move back up to all fours, then bring your buttocks back toward your ankles and lower your forehead down to the ground, curling up into the meditative "child" pose. Stay in this pose for three to five deep breaths. (See Fig. 8.15.) Enjoy the feeling of security and the introspective nature of this position.

8. Lie back down on your stomach in the prone position. Turn your head to one side, with your arms at your sides. Breathe, rest, and enjoy the feeling of tranquillity after giving your spine these tension-relieving stretches. (See Fig. 8.16.)

SITTING SERIES

These exercises can be done either sitting on your mat (legs crossed in tailor position) or in a chair (legs uncrossed, with both

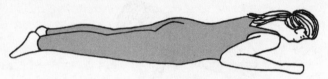

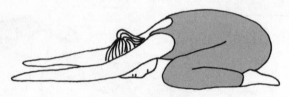

Figure 8.15

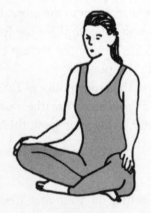

Figure 8.16

feet on the floor). They are excellent stretches to do at work or school when you need a short relaxation break.

1. Start by sitting with your back upright. Feel your spine extending upward and your head balancing on top of your spine. Rest your hands on your lap. Relax your shoulders down, and breathe with full awareness for three to five breaths. (See Fig. 8.17.)

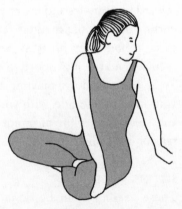

Figure 8.17   Figure 8.18

2. Spinal twist: Place your right hand on your left knee, twist to the left, and look back over your left shoulder. Hold and breathe for three breaths, then untwist, facing front again, and rest. Then switch directions: place your left hand on the right knee, twist to the right, and look over the right shoulder. Hold and breathe for three breaths. Repeat two times. (See Fig. 8.18.)

3. Stretch both arms up overhead, lace your fingers together, then turn your palms outward. Hold this stretch for two deep breaths, and then release your arms and rest. Then stretch your arms out in front of you, lace your fingers, and turn out your palms. Hold for a deep breath, and release. Repeat this stretch with your arms behind your back. (See Figs. 8.19a, 8.19b, and 8.19c.) Stretch luxuriously, the way a cat does, with full extension and awareness.

4. Head/neck: Start with the head nod, moving your chin up and down slowly and gently. Then, with your face forward, tilt your head to the right, moving your right ear toward your right shoulder. Feel the stretch on the left side of your neck. Bring your

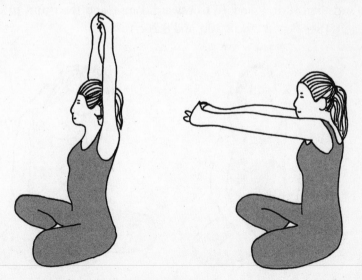

Figure 8.19a   Figure 8.19b

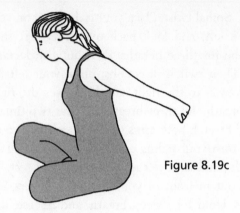

Figure 8.19c

head upright, and then tilt your left ear toward your left shoulder. Feel the stretch on the right side of your neck. Remember to breathe, and move very slowly and gently without any strain as you stretch your neck muscles. With your head upright, turn your face to the right, bringing your chin over toward your right shoulder, without any force or strain. Hold for one deep breath, and then turn your face frontward. Pause, and then turn to the left. (See Figs. 8.20a, 8.20b, and 8.20c.)

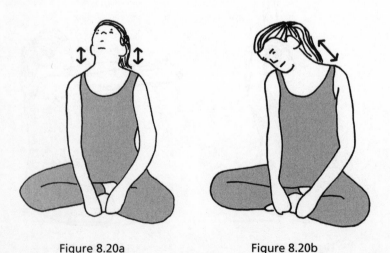

Figure 8.20a   Figure 8.20b

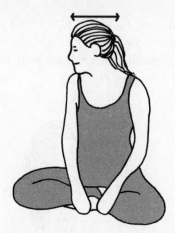

Figure 8.20c

5. Sitting upright, bring your shoulders up to your ears as you inhale deeply through your nose, and then release your shoulders as you breathe out through your mouth with a deep sigh of relief. Repeat this three times, then relax and breathe naturally through your nose. (See Fig. 8.21.)

6. Place your hands on your shoulders and rotate your elbows backward for four rotations. Then circle your elbows forward four times. Focus on the sensation you feel as you fully mobilize your shoulders. (See Fig. 8.22.)

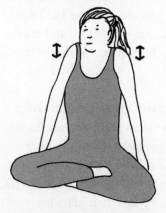

Figure 8.21

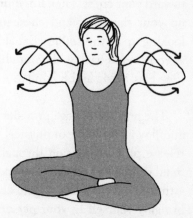

Figure 8.22

7. Stretch your right arm across your chest, and use your left hand to hold and support your right elbow. Hold this stretch for two to three breaths, then release your arm. Repeat this stretch with the left arm. (See Fig. 8.23.)

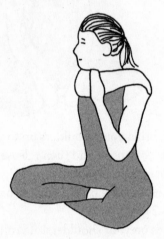

Figure 8.23

8. Cat pose in chair: Place your hands at the back of your chair seat and nod your head downward, bringing your chin toward your chest. Then lift your chin up as you stretch and open up your shoulders and chest, until you are arching backward, looking up at the ceiling. Exhale as you nod forward, and inhale as you stretch back with your chin up. Repeat two to three times. (See Figs. 8.24a and 8.24b.)

The practice of yoga provides stress reduction with the systematic, flowing practice of physical movements and postures. As you release physical tension through body movement, your state of mind is also relieved of its fear and rigidity. Yoga is practiced with an attitude of self-awareness and acceptance. Flexibility develops by bringing yourself to your personal limit, and then allowing your capabilities to expand gently, without force. The HARP yoga series

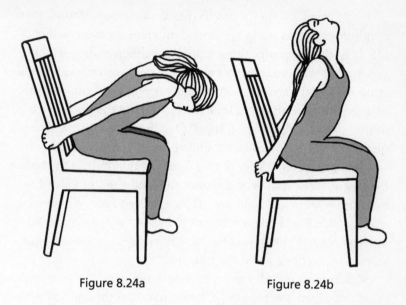

Figure 8.24a   Figure 8.24b

can help you maintain nervous system balance and headache resilience through a daily program of gentle stretching, breathing, and meditation. Yoga is best practiced twice daily. As part of your morning routine, fifteen minutes of yoga helps you start your day with energized muscles and joints, and a gentle attitude. Practiced at the end of the day just before bedtime, yoga relieves accumulated tensions, allowing you to unwind and sleep peacefully.

Focus #3: Mindfulness

Perhaps the most challenging part of taking a relaxation break is to open up to the present moment with all your attention and disregard distracting and critical thoughts. Mindfulness is the term for this awareness in the alert, relaxed state. In his book *Peace Is Every Step*, Vietnamese monk Thich Nhat Hanh instructs, "The miracle is not to walk on water. The miracle is to walk on the green earth in the present moment, to appreciate peace and beauty that are available now."

Participants in our headache reduction groups found that mindfulness breaks made a profound difference in their quality of life. Lois, the mother of three school-age children, described her experience: "Yesterday when I was at the pool with my kids, I put aside my usual parental worries and nagging concerns, and just enjoyed myself with them. I tuned in to the fun they were having in the water and had a good time." One busy executive with frequent tension-type headache smiled broadly when asked if he was being mindful. "Every chance I get I'm mindful, on the train looking out the window at the trees and landscape, or when I get home after work and hold my baby girl close to me. Whenever I walk outside now I take a moment to look up at the sky and take a deep breath. I'm enjoying the time in between headaches now, instead of worrying about the next one."

Mindfulness can also bring freshness and depth to your relationships, when you resolve to "being with" another person with undivided attention. You may take for granted the people with whom you spend the most time. This is poignantly illustrated in Thornton Wilder's play *Our Town*. After Emily dies in childbirth, she is granted one ordinary day to spend with her family. She glories in the delight of common things—the smell of coffee brewing and freshly baked bread. She notices how people can be in the same room, yet not really together or tuned in to one another. Emily pleads, "Oh Mama, just look at me one minute as if I was really here!" In your next interaction with someone, make the effort to truly listen to their words and the inflection in their voice, watch their body language, look into their eyes, and let go of your own thoughts and preconceptions.

Heeding the Signs of Migraine Vulnerability
People with migraines have a fluctuating vulnerability to headaches, a concept called shifting threshold. This means that the likelihood of a headache on any given day varies, and that's why

some days you can sleep late or drink red wine and remain headache free, while other days you take one risky action and you're down with splitting head pain. This shifting threshold, related to the brain's chemical instability, adds to the frustration in identifying consistent patterns or headache triggers.

When you use the HARP techniques of mindfulness and relaxation, you become more aware of your body's fluctuations and can even sense the shifts in your headache threshold. Your body gives you subtle signals that indicate when you are vulnerable to a headache. If you can recognize and tune in to these signals, you can take preventive action, such as avoiding overstimulation, limiting alcohol intake, and getting regular sleep. The signals are unique to each person, and it is only by mindfulness practice that you become aware of your own physiology. Common signals that indicate a lower headache threshold include:

- Sudden fatigue
- A sudden change in appetite, such as carbohydrate craving
- Increasing tension in the neck and shoulders
- Yawning
- Mood changes such as irritability, or feeling "down"
- Becoming sensitive to light or sound
- Experiencing cold extremities
- An intuitive sense that you need to look after yourself and relax

The appropriate response to the signals is to increase your level of self-care. Here are some self-care guidelines:

- Avoid excessive stimulation or excitement.
- Take a break from prolonged activity such as work.
- Stretch the muscles of your neck and back.
- Take a brief period of rest.

- Use your favorite relaxation technique.
- Take a walk or exercise (this counteracts fatigue, increases brain endorphin levels, and reduces headache risk).
- Avoid alcohol and certain foods that may trigger your headaches.

Regular periods of relaxation and mindfulness give you a greater sensitivity to the changes within your body. This is the opposite of what happens when you are chronically engaged in a stress response and focused on external challenges. With the practice of relaxation, you gain the awareness necessary to take the appropriate headache reduction actions.

The HARP Way to Prevent Headaches

- Use a headache log to track headaches and identify triggers.
- Don't skip meals, and avoid foods that trigger your migraines.
- Avoid sensory overload.
- Stick to a regular routine of exercise, rest, and relaxation.

Using the HARP Method That Fits You Best

The HARP methods of breath, body, and mind focus provide you with many different ways to induce relaxation. Experiment with the HARP techniques and find what works best for you at different times of the day and circumstances. Try using any one or a combination of relaxation techniques for at least three consecutive weeks, using your headache log to monitor your success. Don't persist with any method that does not feel "right" for you.

When you are under extreme time pressure, a minute of breathing diaphragmatically or doing a few yoga stretches are quick stress relievers. A mindful walk around the neighborhood in the evening is a good way to relieve the stress of a sedentary day. Sitting by a window and meditating in the morning, before starting your day's activities, will have a carryover effect throughout the day, making you more stress-hardy, efficient, and aware.

The more you practice the HARP techniques, the more easily and quickly you will relax. As you gain greater sensitivity to your personal state of stress, you will discover that your body instinctively "knows" which techniques will make you feel better. With continued practice, the responses you have learned—to take some deep, slow breaths, stretch those tense muscles, and stop the negative cycle of thoughts—will become second nature to you. You will have mastered the HARP way to prevent headaches—naturally.

9

Self-Care for Well-Being:
Beyond Headache Reduction

As children, we wake up with excitement and anticipation about the day ahead. Remember the first day of summer vacation, or a special birthday? As an adult, how often do you feel that spontaneous passion about life, about where you're going to be that day, who you are going to be with, and what you will encounter? As you use the HARP relaxation techniques more and more in your daily life, you will find that the benefits of the relaxation response extend well beyond the reduction in your headaches. By countering stress-mode functioning with mindful awareness, you become more attuned to your own natural functioning and the rhythm of the world around you. Moreover, your vitality improves as you remove the major obstacles to healthy function—chronic stress, nervous system overload, and poor self-care practices.

This chapter describes some of the additional benefits you will gain from the HARP program, including:

- Stress hardiness
- Creativity
- Optimism and attunement
- Self-awareness and improved self-care

Stress Hardiness

Health is more than the absence of disease; it's living with exuberance, with joy and optimism in being alive and part of the world around you. There is a spiritual dimension to health that involves your concepts of who you are and why you're here, what you value most, and how you find meaning in your life. In studies of executives in high-stress positions, researcher Suzanne Kobasa discovered that the healthiest employees shared certain "stress-hardy" attitudes, called the 3 Cs. Stress-hardy executives saw problems as *challenges* to learn from, maintained faith in their capability to intervene and take *control* when necessary, and felt a sense of *commitment* to their jobs and coworkers.

When you have a chronic condition like migraine, you don't always wake up glad to be alive. It's not easy to feel a sense of control when you're the victim of recurrent head pain that can occur without warning, seemingly without cause, to disturb your life and defeat your ability to function. How do you regain a sense of control in those circumstances? How can you view your migraines as a challenge and the pain as a reminder to take better care of yourself and become more committed to your health and well-being?

One headache clinic patient, an elementary-school teacher, shook her head with sadness and resignation when the group discussed stress hardiness. Evelyn had migraines two or three times a week, and suffered from fibromyalgia and irritable bowel syndrome. Her fourth-grade class this year was very difficult, and she felt little support from the administration or parents. Her job no longer held any pleasure or satisfaction for her, and she was counting the days until retirement. We all sympathized with her situation, acknowledging the enormous responsibility teachers carry, and how chronic pain gnawing on her nerves would make the job a struggle every day. Simply by expressing her predicament and sense of frustration to the group, Evelyn had taken an important self-care step. She began to think of her problem as a challenge; her work situation was impacting her health and had to be dealt with in order to break the stress–tension–pain cycle she was in. The numerous preventative medications and pain relievers she took daily were not sufficient; they did not get to the root of the problem, to what generated such tension and anxiety. Self-care action was necessary.

Everyone noticed the change when Evelyn came back to class a few weeks later, smiling and eager to share the self-care action she had taken. She had written a letter to her administrator stating her case—considering her age and twenty-five years of loyal service to the school, and the medical conditions she had that are exacerbated by stress, she requested fairness and input in setting up her class for next year. Instead of giving up and feeling utterly powerless, she chose to do something about her dilemma, and that step alone made her feel better. She felt she had been heard, and had found some way to exert control of her situation.

Here are other examples of self-care actions that HARP participants told us about that made a big difference in decreasing headaches and enhancing their quality of life:

- After arriving home from work, Sandy routinely heads to the sunroom to take twenty minutes alone to sit and meditate before starting dinner and other household tasks.
- Chris uses the time when her toddler's on a playdate to listen to relaxation audiotapes.
- Terry requested an adjustment in his work schedule to avoid frequent shift changes that disturbed his regular sleep cycles and triggered migraines.
- Sara has set up a routine time to work on her favorite hobby and signed up for a yoga class.
- Alex dropped a second part-time job, after recognizing that the extra money was not worth the added stress.
- Pat set up her office computer to display an hourly reminder to take a three-minute break to stretch, breathe, and shake off tension.

In every HARP group we ran, we saw that to gain control of one's migraines, a major change in attitude was mandatory. Once people accepted their headaches as a recurring condition, they decided they may as well learn how best to live with them. They began to view their migraines as a challenge in their lives rather than as a personal sign of failure. Our patients always felt such a sense of relief once they understood that their nervous system's sensitivity to change was part of what migraineurs inherit along with the headaches. They were motivated to regain control—to make choices in their day-to-day life that helped maintain nervous system balance and would enhance both resilience to stress and resistance to headaches. They made a commitment to self-care, to being actively involved in preventing their migraines and enhancing their health and well-being.

Changing the Things You Can Control

Take a look at your life and make a list of your stressors, situations that cause you frustration, anger, or anxiety. These stressors are no doubt affecting your health, and you need to deal with them if you want to be healthy. Take them one at a time. Look at what aspects are out of your control, but also look carefully to see what aspects can be changed, eliminated, or adjusted. Be inspired by Reinhold Niebuhr's *Serenity Prayer:* "Grant me the serenity to accept the things I cannot change, the courage to change the things I can, and the wisdom to know the difference."

The Five Ls of Success: Learn, Labor, Love, Laughter, and Letting Go

Consider the "Five Ls of Success," described by Dr. Barry Greiff of Harvard Business School, as a tool you can use to examine your life and see if all the ingredients are there to be happy and fulfilled, for health that goes beyond symptom relief. Spend a few minutes considering these questions, and ask yourself if any of the five Ls are missing.

Learn: Do you look at each day as an opportunity to learn, to increase your knowledge of yourself and the world? Learning keeps you vibrant and alive. Studies show that the power of learning stimulates the brain and keeps it functioning properly, with memory intact. If you read every day, listen to news, enroll in a course, or keep up-to-date with your profession, you will be healthier. Look at your life right now—is learning an important priority?

Labor: Do you have something you work on each day that utilizes your special interests, talents, and skills? It's been said that people shouldn't worry about what the world needs. Instead, do the work that makes you come alive, because fully alive, vibrant individuals are what the world needs most. What do you like best about your work? Can your work situation be improved? Do you need to make any changes to become more fulfilled and committed to your job?

Love: Dean Ornish, M.D., has become famous for his bestselling books on living with heart disease. Although he is mostly associated with prescribing a heart-healthy diet, he firmly believes that human connections are a critical element in living a long, healthy life. Do your relationships bring out the best in you and them? Do you have people with whom you can regularly share joys and sorrows? Remember, "A joy shared is doubled, a sorrow shared is halved." When you spend time with loved ones, is it time when you are mindfully living "in the moment"?

Laughter: In *Anatomy of an Illness as Perceived by the Patient,* Norman Cousins relates how he took a proactive approach to dealing with his chronic debilitating illness. He resolved to test his hypothesis that if bad feelings and distressing emotions have the ability to make one ill, then a positive emotion, like humor, has the power to make one healthy. After discussing his ideas with his doctor, he prescribed two hours of laughter every day as part of his hospital treatment. A special blood test that measures inflammatory response—the sedimentation rate—was taken before and after two-hour sessions of watching funny TV shows or reading joke books. These tests showed a lowered sedimentation rate post-laughter that was still down before the next day's laughter treatment. Cousins became one of the small minority of people who overcame his illness. He attributed his recovery largely to his determination to take charge of his health care and to the healing power of humor. Do you make sure laughter is a regular part of your day? Do you spend time with people who are easy to laugh with, include a comedy with your video/ DVD rentals, keep books or audiotapes of favorite comedians on hand?

Letting go: Stress inhibits our ability to let go. The stressed-out mind becomes trapped in negative thoughts and dire predictions, and one's attitude becomes overly critical and despairing. Use relaxation techniques to give yourself a break from worries and anxieties, and strengthen and restore your ability to cope. Any activity done with mindful focus—taking a walk, breathing, stretching—is an antidote to the stress response. When you let go and take time out for a relaxation break, your mind is freed from routine worrying and you can feel an expansion in ideas, thoughts, and feelings. How often do you take time for yourself, letting go of responsibilities for just a little while? Do you journal, play an instrument, listen to music, sing, or create art? Time for letting go must become a priority in your life, as it restores the balance and energy you need to weather life's ups and downs.

Creativity

When stressed, your automatically narrowed focus of attention makes challenges appear overwhelming. When you relax, you can see beyond your own immediate needs. This relaxed state allows different parts of the brain, called association areas, to connect with one another. It is in this relaxed state that creative ideas and thoughts flow most readily.

Thomas Edison, arguably the greatest inventor of all time, used relaxation periods such as naps when working on a problem. He would get back to work refreshed and inspired with creative solutions.

We know how hard it is to overcome a "block" when trying to solve a problem such as trying to recall a fact. The harder we try, the more frustrated we become; the more stressed we become the more elusive the answer.

Meditation is useful when you need to think "outside the box" to solve a problem and create solutions. When stuck on a problem (such as trying to make a difficult decision), take a "time-out." Mentally acknowledge the problem, briefly run through your list of pros and cons, and acknowledge the work you have already put into solving it. Then wrap it up and give the package over to your creative mind, saying "Here you are, you do it now!" Begin the relaxation response with focused breathing, counting or repeating your mantra with each outbreath. Ignore the problem if it comes up (it will almost certainly do so, as thoughts intrude on your relaxation) and go back to your focused breathing. After five to ten minutes, get up, stretch, and enjoy the new ideas and creative thoughts that come to you during the day. This technique also helps prevent accumulating stress and frustration from triggering a migraine.

Journaling Your Troubles Away

Writing is another way to calm your mind when it's wound up and whirring away with distracting thoughts. Rachel Naomi Remen, M.D., who holds poetry workshops with cancer survivors at Commonweal in California, is convinced about the healing power of writing. In her preface to a book that explores this concept, *Poetic Medicine*, Remen says, "One of the best-kept secrets in this technically oriented culture is that simply speaking truth heals. . . . Recovering the poet strengthens the healer and sets free the unique song that is at the heart of every life."

James Pennebaker has done clinical research to examine the effects of journaling on the immune system. He divided a cohort of college students into three groups: one group wrote about the things that bothered or mattered to them, the second group kept a diary of superficial daily routines, and the third group did not journal at all. There was a significant difference in the group who journaled about their concerns; they had fewer clinic visits and healthier blood test results.

Journal Writing Instructions: Start by setting aside fifteen minutes a day, and simply sitting down and writing nonstop. Don't edit, correct your spelling, or make cross-outs. Give yourself permission to write down whatever you are thinking about. Freely express any feeling that comes up while you write, particularly ones like anger, fear, or sadness that you often bottle up or are too inhibited to tell anyone about. Don't write in a fancy journal, or imagine you're penning an autobiography that someone will read someday. Make yourself the only audience. Try writing on a few sheets of loose-leaf paper, and remember that you can tear it up when you're through to make sure no one else will ever see it! It's the process of writing and freely expressing your mind that is healing in this exercise. Try journaling at bedtime, to clear your mind of the day's trials and tribulations. And, if you ever wake up in the middle of the night and can't sleep due to your anxious, racing thoughts, sit down and journal until you are relaxed and breathing easily again.

Optimism and Attunement

Stress and pain can be isolating. During a migraine, you may feel alone, alienated, and withdrawn. When assailed by the stress of pain, thinking becomes negative and you expect the worst. The body rejects positive ideas when the sympathetic nervous system is actively engaged in responding to stress. You automatically think, "This headache will never end!" or even "I'm going to die."

Breaking the cycle of negative thinking is a hidden benefit of using relaxation methods to prevent headache. Once you relax, you become receptive to healing and life-enhancing thoughts. You also become more aware of life and the natural world around you. *Attunement* is the term for this feeling of belonging or connecting with life. It represents an expansion of awareness, in contrast to the contraction that occurs with stress. This is a wonderful experience. It may not happen often but, when it does, it is clearly the source of true optimism. At this moment, we feel truly alive and are able to accept this experience without having to intellectualize or rationalize it.

Using Guided Imagery to Lighten Your Load

The following exercise gives you an opportunity to relax deeply and use your imagination to regain a positive attitude about that part of you that often causes you such aggravation—your headaches.

> Lie down or sit back comfortably in a chair, and allow yourself to relax. Gently, and without judgment, scan your body, breathing in to each part, starting with your feet, bringing in healing oxygen and energy, release and comfort. Breathe out

tension and discomfort as you exhale. Moving upward, progressively relax your legs, arms, abdomen, chest, back, shoulders, and neck.

Now gently focus on your head. Breathe in and feel the energy gently circulating in your head. Become aware of your scalp. Relax and soften the muscles in your scalp. Relax the skin, vessels, and nerves. Breathe in soothing oxygen. Soften the muscles of your face, around your eyes, mouth, lips, jaw, ears, and chin. Feel relaxation deepening, penetrating deep into your head and into your brain. You are allowing the brain waves to slow down, without any effort, just by relaxing, taking a well-deserved break. Constantly on the go, your brain appreciates a rest from time to time. It functions more efficiently in a peaceful state.

Now see if you can visualize your brain, there inside your head. What is the color, the texture, and the weight of it? Visualize the nerve cells, smoothly firing off messages, coordinating every movement, whether conscious or unconscious, doing everything that needs to be done to keep you alive and functioning in healthy balance, smoothly, efficiently, amazingly! You smile to yourself, realizing perhaps that you haven't given this wonderful, valuable brain the recognition that it deserves.

Breathe deeply, allowing a fresh supply of oxygen to revitalize every nerve cell. Enjoy breathing deeply and fully for several breaths. Rest, relax, and rejuvenate your brain. Of course there are times when you feel less than loving toward your head and your brain. Sometimes you've felt aggravated and frustrated by the headaches that can be so painful and disruptive in your life. However, it's important to pay attention to your headaches and use pain as a signal: stop and ask yourself how you can take better care of yourself? Think about this now, tune in to the wise health adviser within you, and listen to what your body tells you.

Now take some time to think about your headaches. What changes do you visualize in your head and brain when a headache occurs? What image comes to mind? Think about it while staying completely relaxed. Allow an image of your headache to emerge. Let the image become clear and vivid, and observe it carefully. What do you smell, taste, hear, feel as the headache comes on? What is it that represents the problem? What happens as the pain builds up in your head?

When you know this, let another image appear that represents healing, the resolution of the headache. Again, simply allow it to arise spontaneously and observe this image well, from different perspectives. What is it about this image that represents healing and relief of headache pain? Continue breathing deeply and fully while you vividly imagine your head and brain free of pain, functioning easily and in perfect health.

Now, recall the headache image along with the healing, pain-relief image, and consider the two together. How do they relate to each other? Which is larger, more powerful? If the image of the headache is more powerful, see if you can change that. Imagine the healing image becoming stronger, more powerful, more vivid. Imagine the healthy, pain-free head to be much larger and much more powerful than the headache. Continue to breathe calmly and rhythmically. Remember that whenever you feel a headache coming on, you can rest, relax, and use this healing imagery to help yourself obtain relief.

A Personal View of Migraine: Donna's Healing Headache Imagery

I see my brain like a big heavy gray cloud in my head, dark and threatening, flashes of lightning and rumbles of thunder, sounds getting louder, lights more glaring and obtrusive. The cloud becomes heavier, slower, and darker as the headache advances, from gray to black. My mood darkens too. I feel the pressure it creates in my head, the tension and congestion in my face. I feel sad, and the pressure and pain build up inside until I begin to cry; my tears are like the rain falling.

After a while, I begin to feel a change in the atmosphere. The clouds are moving now, they're lifting up, getting lighter and higher in the sky, and they're moving away. I feel this movement and my spirit begins to lift. My headaches feel like the clouds, not solid and immobile, but full of energy and movement. And eventually, there's a beam of light breaking through the clouds. It's the sun! As the sky brightens and the storm clouds move on, I begin to feel hopeful and relieved that the storm is ending. The whole world is becoming lighter and brighter and fresher. My head gradually feels light and easy; my mood becomes clear and calm. I see colors more vividly; the grass is greener than ever. I feel a refreshing breeze on my face, cooling my forehead, drying my tears, soothing and gentle, and I breathe easily. Let go and relax. The storm's over, and I'm grateful. I have survived it once again.

Self-Awareness, Improved Self-Care . . . A Healthier World

When stress becomes chronic, body feeling is dampened and reduced. You lose sense of what your body tells you and ignore the signals to rest, retreat, and regroup. Putting the needs of others first, you shortchange your own needs. When this becomes a habit, you run the risk of becoming depleted and "burned out."

Periods of relaxation not only reduce the risk of burnout, but also lead to greater self-respect. The combination of self-awareness and self-respect is essential to self-care. This growth in awareness is evident in HARP participants who gradually learn to recognize the signals of an impending migraine. They learn to avoid headache triggers (like skipping that glass of wine with dinner, or postponing that trip to the mall) and take special care of themselves when they sense their headache threshold is low.

With the growing awareness that comes from periods of regular relaxation and mindfulness, you will find that your diet becomes healthier, your work becomes more efficient, and your relationships more satisfying. This is born out of the true respect for life that you will discover when you respect your core needs and values. This awareness eventually extends from yourself to others, as you gain the health and vitality necessary to support and nurture the life of your family and community.

10

Staying with the HARP:
Preventing Relapses

It doesn't take very long before you experience positive results from using the HARP relaxation techniques. In our weekly Headache Reduction Program, it is usually by the third week that most people report some benefit—either a feeling of reestablishing some control over headaches, a diminishing headache frequency, or other spin-off benefits such as improved sleep, more self-awareness, and a greater sense of control.

The mutual support of participants in the group and the energy of the shared atmosphere encourage initial rapid progress. For many, experiencing the Relaxation Response provides a strong contrast to ongoing cycles of stress, tension, headache, and more stress. This initial positive phase lasts for a few months after the six weekly group sessions end.

With the passage of time, group participants may lapse in using their relaxation methods. The loss of the support of the group, erosion of the initial enthusiasm, and lapsing into old habits are some of the reasons why they go back to their old ways.

You, the individual reader, do not have the "jumpstart" of the group—that initial burst of energy and enthusiasm of being a participant in a headache reduction group. In the end, this does not matter. Sustained benefits from using relaxation methods depend on whether you persevere and keep practicing.

Perseverance is vital to eventual success in trying to control headaches using the tools you have learned. What happens if you do not continue trying to integrate relaxation into your daily routine? You may end up where you started with:

- Frequent headaches
- Dependency on analgesics with the risk of rebound headaches
- Potential side effects from medication
- Discouragement and frustration
- The negative cycle of stress–tension–headache

Your Body Remembers

You have learned about the biological basis for migraine and that it is a "package deal." This package includes an enhanced responsiveness or sensitivity of the nervous system.

You have learned about treatment options and have acquired new tools to manage headaches and to avoid or prevent migraine attacks. The HARP exercises raise your migraine threshold and protect your nervous system from overload.

The real treasure and benefit from using the HARP techniques lies in your actual experience—what you have felt in your body, mind, and spirit when you relax. Just reading about it or intellectualizing is not sufficient. Once you have learned to relax, you can recall the experience of relaxation at will. Your body remembers what it is like to disengage the sympathetic drive; it stores and encodes the experience of relaxation in the nervous system. You will find that just by taking that initial deep diaphragmatic breath in response to a stressful situation, your body will follow the cue to relax, let go of muscle tension, and calm down.

Old Habits Die Hard

Keeping up a regular practice of relaxation or de-stressing techniques takes commitment. Ideally, you would attend refresher classes and remain in touch with others who are trying to do the same thing. Similarly, you would have the encouragement and support of those closest to you. Many headache sufferers look for support from outside sources such as books, audiotapes, Internet groups, and support groups. These are helpful, but ultimately the drive comes from within yourself as you seek to maintain and restore a healthy balance in your life.

Participants in the HARP groups planned to hold reunions, asked for refresher courses, and set up e-mail links. Although they started out with good intentions, they found that relaxation practices can become lost in the pressures of life. It's important to recognize the obstacles that can challenge your ability to stay on the headache reduction pathway:

- *Old habits.* Changing habits and mental attitudes requires regular practice and time. It is normal to resist change. Shear inertia often pulls us back to old ways.
- *Stress.* The negative cycle of stress and time pressure can lead you to forego periods of self-care. Day-to-day stress can rob you of your contact or attunement with the gentle feeling of deep relaxation. You can lose this feeling if you do not periodically take relaxation breaks or nurture and protect your self-care practice.
- *Frustration.* Remember that the tendency to migraine is biologically determined. There is no quick fix; nor is there an absolutely foolproof way to prevent all headaches. If you forget this, you may give up on relaxation practice and lapse back into the cycle of negative thinking and stress.

Keep Relaxation Fresh

HARP's success in preventing migraines lies in the regular practice of the relaxation techniques. A good way to counteract the risk of your practice becoming stale is to vary the techniques—or "mix it up." Different variations and combinations of relaxation methods are all effective. Experimenting with different HARP techniques will allow you to identify what works best and in what circumstances. For example, when you wake up in the morning feeling anxious about the day, start by enjoying a "mindful" shower: focus on the heat of the water warming your muscles, the delightful smell of the soap or shampoo as you lather up, and inhale the soothing steam. If you don't have time for a twenty-minute yoga routine or meditation, then do five minutes of stretching. Remember that even short breaks throughout the day prevent headaches. Taking four deep breaths with awareness while waiting for the traffic light to turn green, or while standing in line at the grocery store, will effectively keep your body from accumulating stress.

If the day ends and you realize that you have not done any relaxation techniques, it is not too late. Doing a body scan or breathing rhythmically as you count backward will help you release the stress of the day and lull you to sleep naturally.

Here are some of the techniques to choose from with examples of how you may use them:

Breathing Techniques

• *Diaphragmatic breathing:* Start with a deep breath in through the nose, and breathe out through your mouth with a deep sigh; then continue breathing in and out through your nose. Soften your neck, shoulders, chest, and abdomen, and breathe fully and rhythmically, letting go of any muscle tension with each breath. Watch how your belly expands on inhalation and contracts as you breathe out. Enhance your mental focus by counting or repeating a mantra with each exhalation. Use this technique in stressful situations or emergencies, such as during a headache, when stuck in traffic, or just before a business meeting or presentation.

Body Techniques

• *Gentle stretching:* Use the simple stretching exercises you learned from the HARP yoga series. Clasp your fingers together, stretch your arms above your head, in front of you, and then back behind you. Breathe, and focus on the sensation of stretching your muscles. Bring your shoulders up to your ears, then release them down. Gently stretch your neck muscles: rotate your head slowly from left to right, then nod your head, lifting the chin up and bending the head down. Use this technique at work or at home to break up developing muscle tension.

• *Regular rhythmic exercise:* Schedule regular periods of exercise into your week, such as a twenty-minute walk at lunchtime. Whenever you feel restless or anxious and have difficulty sitting still, get up and stretch or go for a short stroll.

• *Daily yoga:* Practice the HARP yoga series for ten to twenty minutes. The best times are after your morning shower when your muscles are warmed up and at the end of the day to release tension and promote sleep. Practice yoga at least three or four times a week. In addition to yoga, try other forms of pleasurable exercise such as walking, biking, swimming, and working out at the gym.

• *Short "minute" breaks:* Take short stretch breaks throughout the day, at least once an hour when sitting at your desk or computer, and whenever you are waiting—at the grocery store, at the train station, or by a fax machine. In the evening when watching television, get on the floor and do some yoga stretching during commercial breaks.

Mind Techniques

• *Visualization or guided imagery:* Recalling a peaceful or favorite place, like a tropical beach or your grandmother's kitchen, gives you a mental "time-out" and allows you to enjoy the same positive and mental physical reactions as being there. Use this technique when you are feeling low or blue, are having difficulty sleeping, or recovering from a headache.

• *Self-expression with journal writing:* Write down whatever is on your mind at least once a week, allowing your thoughts to flow freely (without editing) for fifteen to twenty minutes. Writing can be useful before bedtime to release pent-up emotions or worries, or if you wake up and cannot sleep due to distressing thoughts.

• *Mindfulness:* Live with awareness of the present moment, opening all your senses to what surrounds you. Do this whenever you can, particularly during mealtimes, during social interactions, and while driving your car. Take advantage of transitions between activities by taking deep, refreshing breaths before you enter your home or workplace.

Useful Reminders

There are many creative ways to remind yourself to take time out of your busy day for self-care.

• A note in your diary or calendar is a good place to start. Even the icon of a smiley face to remind you to practice some aspect of headache prevention is helpful.

• At work, choose computer screensavers with soothing images or sounds, such as virtual ocean waves or a mountain stream. You can also program your computer to give you hourly reminders to take relaxation breaks.

• When you gaze at photographs of special vacations or happy events, you experience the same pleasurable emotions as when you were there. A picture of the beach, a memorable sunset, or a view from a hilltop also serves as a reminder to take a few deep breaths during the day.

• Making an appointment with yourself is a very useful way to set aside time for your own self-care. Write it into your appointment calendar at least once a week. Schedule a massage, an afternoon picnic lunch by yourself, or a meditative walk at your favorite park.

• Keeping a headache log serves not only to identify headache triggers and patterns of frequency, but will also remind you to keep practicing self-care techniques. An increase in the number of headaches will be your signal to examine whether you are getting regular sleep, exercise, meals, and relaxation breaks.

Outside Help

At times you may feel alone and isolated in dealing with your headaches. You may feel that people who don't get migraines can never understand what it's like to have chronically recurring headaches and how distressing it is to live in anticipation of the next one.

This feeling of isolation can make it difficult to persevere on the self-care path to headache control. You can break out of your isolation by drawing on outside help offered by professionals who are dedicated to migraine education and relief of headache. Headache support groups and the therapeutic alliance with your health-care provider are important sources of outside help.

A Healing Partnership

Remember that migraines are a medical condition. Don't expect yourself to diagnose and treat migraines alone. A mutually respectful relationship with a health-care practitioner may be necessary for optimal headache control. Practicing the HARP self-care techniques will complement and strengthen the medical care you receive.

Headache Specialty Organizations

There are national organizations that specialize in migraine education and support; they can also help you find local support groups.

National Headache Foundation (NHF)
428 West St. James Place, 2nd floor
Chicago, IL 60614 -2750
Telephone: 888-NHF-5552
www.headaches.org

American Council for Headache Education (ACHE)
19 Mantua Road
Mount Royal, NJ 08061
Telephone: 856-423-0258 or 800-255-ACHE (2243)
www.achenet.org

National Migraine Association (MAGNUM)
113 South Saint Asaph, Suite 300
Alexandria, VA 22314
Telephone: 703-739-9384
www.migraines.org

A Final Word of Encouragement

Medical science has come a long way in understanding the migraine disorder—knowledge about the neurochemical origins of migraine is gradually replacing the old prejudicial notion that headaches are caused by a personality deficiency or the inability to handle stress. As medical research uncovers the genetic and biological secrets of migraine, newer and more effective therapies are being developed. But you don't have to suffer while waiting for the "perfect" migraine drug. With daily practice of the HARP self-care techniques, you can reduce the pain and impact of your headaches naturally and, what is more, enhance your vitality, well-being, and your resiliency to stress.

Glossary of Terms

Acetylcholine: The principal neurotransmitter of the parasympathetic nervous system.

Alarm reaction: The initial response to threat. Described by Hans Selye in 1936.

Alternative medicine: Medical practices that have not yet been scientifically validated.

Analgesic: A remedy used to relieve pain.

Antidepressant: A drug used to improve depressed mood.

Aura: The sensory disturbance (usually visual) that precedes the headache of the migraine. This may occur in isolation (known as a migraine equivalent) or precede the headache (migraine with aura).

Autogenics: A system of progressively relaxing different muscle groups in turn.

Autonomic nervous system: The involuntary nervous system.

Awareness: Perception in consciousness.

Biofeedback: Formal technique of learning to induce the Relaxation Response by responding to measured body signals (using instruments that monitor temperature, muscle tension, or brain wave activity).

Biological core: The concept of the central source of energy in the body—collectively, the autonomic and cardiovascular system. Eastern philosophies view this as the body center of chi (dantien) or, in yoga, the chakra.

Biological trait: A physical and physiological characteristic that may or may not have genetic basis.

Body scan: A relaxation exercise in which awareness is focused on different parts of the body, searching out hidden points of tension.

Cognitive distortion: Wrong thinking that has different causes and results in more stress.

Comorbidity: Medical conditions that coexist more frequently than expected.

Contact: Awareness coupled with excitation and feeling. We can make contact with our own self, nature, or each other.

Diaphragmatic breathing: Use of the diaphragm in breathing to promote relaxation. Also known as belly breathing.

Endorphins: Literally meaning "endogenous morphine." These are some of the natural chemicals produced in the brain to suppress pain.

Enhanced responsiveness: The increased reactivity or sensitivity of the nervous system that accompanies the migraine trait.

Ergotamine: A drug derived from rye fungus. This was one of the first drugs used to treat acute migraine headache.

Fibromyalgia: A medical condition characterized by chronic pain and muscle spasms. Fibromyalgia is more common in migraine sufferers than expected.

Fight-or-flight response: The changes in the body resulting from activation of the sympathetic nervous system in response to threat.

Gene: The DNA sequence that is translated into the synthesis of a specific protein.

Genetic predisposition: The inherited tendency to certain physiological and disease states, such as migraine.

Habituation: The lessening of response with repeated stimulus.

The lack of habituation in migraine sufferers is an element of the enhanced responsiveness of the nervous system.

HARP: The Headache Reduction Program on which this book is based.

Headache: A pain in the head. There are many causes.

Hemicrania: The Greek term for "half a head." It is an alternative term for a migraine headache.

Hippocampus: This part of the brain, which looks like a seahorse, is vital to memory.

Homeostasis: The maintenance of stable body function. This term, introduced by Claude Bernard (known as the father of physiology), comes from the Greek *homios,* meaning similar, and *stasis,* the ability to remain the same.

Inflammation: The change in the tissues with increased blood flow, warmth, swelling, and pain. Release of chemicals induces inflammation in migraine.

Learned helplessness: A dire consequence of stress where we feel unable to control the outcome. It is a state that precedes giving up.

Letdown headache: A headache following reduction in stress or upon relaxation, such as weekends. This is common in migraine.

Limbic system: The emotional part of the brain.

Magnetic resonance spectroscopy: A diagnostic technique using high-intensity magnetic fields to determine the chemical composition of tissues. This tool has been used to study migraine.

Meditation: Deep relaxation with focused awareness. There are many techniques of meditation.

Migraine: A biological disorder the intermittent expression of which is headache.

Migraine equivalent: The migraine aura occurring without a headache.

Migraine generator: That term given to the groups of nerve cells deep in the brain thought to generate the impulses of a migraine attack.

Migraine threshold: The degree of vulnerability to a migraine attack. The lower the threshold, the easier it is to get a migraine.

Migraineur: The European term for a migraine sufferer.

Mindfulness: Awareness in the relaxed state.

Mysticism: The interpretation of emotional and physical sensations as coming from an outside source such as a higher power.

Natural rhythm: The normal rate of natural living function such as breathing.

Neuron: A nerve cell with defined chemical and electrical properties.

Neurophysiological: The workings of a healthy nervous system.

Neurotransmitter: The chemical messenger released by one nerve cell across a synapse onto another nerve cell.

Norepinephrine: The principal neurotransmitter of the sympathetic nervous system.

Parasympathetic nervous system: The part of the involuntary nervous system that is engaged in relaxation, digestion, or pleasure.

Perception: The feeling or sensation that forms the basis of awareness.

Photophobia: Sensitivity to light that is usually part of a migraine attack. The word means "afraid of light."

Postdrome: The state of being that follows a migraine attack.

Prodrome: The change in well-being that precedes the symptoms of a migraine attack. This is analogous to the atmospheric changes of a developing storm.

Progressive muscle relaxation: The systematic tightening and relaxation of muscle groups to induce relaxation.

Prophylaxis: The prevention of disease or disorder.

Psychoneuroimmunology: A new medical term for the study of how the mind, emotions, and immune system influence each other.

Psychosomatic: Physical symptoms or disorders that result from mental or emotional causes.

Rebound headache: The recurrence of headache due to withdrawal from an analgesic. Rebound headaches are unique to migraine sufferers.

Relapse: Returning to old bad habits or a recurrence of a disorder or disease.

Relaxation response: The opposite of the stress response.

Resilience: Strength and resistance to threat, challenge, and disease.

Rest: A state of relaxation in which physical, emotional, and mental activity are reduced.

Self-care: Rational safeguarding of one's own health and vitality. This is an essential aspect of migraine prevention.

Serotonin: This neurotransmitter is widely distributed througout the brain and is involved in many functions. Levels of serotonin are unstable in migraine and depleted in depression.

Shifting threshold: The varying level of vulnerability to disorder. This accounts for why migraine may be activated by a certain trigger at one time but not another.

Side effect: An undesirable effect of medication.

Sonophobia: Sensitivity to sound. This often accompanies the migraine.

SSRI: An antidepressant that acts specifically on increasing serotonin levels at the synapse.

Stress: A term commonly used to describe the body's response to emotional and physical challenges. In essence, it is the response of adaptation to change.

Stressor: The emotional or physical challenge that induces the stress response.

Sympathetic nervous system: The part of the involuntary nervous system that responds to stress.

Synapse: The junction and point of communication between nerve cells and their processes.

Tension: A prolonged low-grade stress response.

Tension headache: A nondisabling pressing headache. Migraine sufferers often have this type of headache in addition to their migraines.

Transformed migraine: The progression of migraine pattern from occasional severe headache to headaches occurring at least 50 percent of the time.

Trigger: The event or stimulus that evokes a particular migraine attack.

Triptan: A new class of drugs designed specifically for the treatment of migraine headache. These have largely replaced the ergotamines.

Yoga: The Eastern discipline of mindfulness and systematic relaxation. There are many types of yoga.

Additional Reading

Here are several helpful books grouped in broad categories:

Historical Aspect of Migraine

Liveing, E. *On Megrim, Sick-Headache and Some Allied Disorders: A Contribution to the Pathology of Nerve-Storms.* London: J. and A. Churchill, 1873.

Wolff, H.G. *Wolff's Headache and Other Head Pain.* 2nd ed. New York: Oxford University Press, 1963.

Technical and Medically Based Books

Rapoport, A. E., Sheftell, F. D., and Purdy, R. A. *Advanced Therapy of Headache.* Ontario: B. C. Decker Inc., 1999.

Saper, J. R., Silberstein, S. D., Gordon, C. D., Hamel, R. L., and Swidan, S. *Handbook of Headache Management. A Practical Guide to Diagnosis and Treatment of Head, Neck, and Facial Pain.* 2nd ed. Baltimore: Lippincott Williams and Wilkins, 1999.

Silberstein, S. D., Lipton, R. B., and Goadsby, P. J. *Headache in Clinical Practice.* London: Martin Dunitz, 2002.

Books Written for the Headache Sufferer

Buchholz, D. *Heal Your Headache: The 1-2-3 Program for Taking Charge of Your Pain.* New York: Workman Publishing, 2002.

Cady, R., and Farmer, K. *Headache Free. A Personalized Program to Stop*

Migraine, Cluster, Sinus, Tension, Menstrual and Rebound Headaches. New York: Bantam Books, 1996.

Diamond, S., and Diamond, M. L. *Contemporary Diagnosis and Management of Headache and Migraine.* Newtown, Penn.: Handbooks in Health Care Company, 2000.

Sacks, O. *Migraine: Understanding a Common Disorder.* Berkeley: University of California Press, 1985.

Stress Management and Relaxation Techniques

Anderson, B. *Stretching at Your Computer or Desk.* Bolinas, Calif.: Shelter Publications, 1997.

Benson, H. *The Relaxation Response.* New York: William Morrow, 1975.

Benson, H. *Beyond the Relaxation Response.* New York: Times Books, 1984.

Benson, H., and Stewart, E. M. *The Wellness Book. The Comprehensive Guide to Maintaining Health and Treating Stress-Related Illness.* New York: Simon & Schuster, 1992.

Borysenko, J. *Minding the Body, Mending the Mind.* Reading, Mass.: Addison-Wesley, 1987.

Burns, D. *The Feeling Good Handbook.* New York: Plume, 1989.

Carrico, M., and *Yoga Journal*, eds. *Yoga Basics: The Essential Beginner's Guide to Yoga for a Lifetime of Health and Fitness.* New York: Henry Holt, 1997.

Cousins, N. *Anatomy of an Illness as Perceived by the Patient.* New York: Bantam Books, 1981.

Fox, J. *Poetic Medicine.* New York: Tarcher/Putnam, 1997.

Gawain, S. *Creative Visualization.* New York: Bantam Books, 1978.

Hanh, T. N. *Peace Is Every Step: The Path of Mindfulness in Everyday Life.* New York: Bantam Books, 1976.

Kabat-Zinn, J. *Full Catastrophe Living. Using the Wisdom of Your Body and Mind to Face Stress and Pain.* New York: Delacorte Press, 1990.

Mason, L. J. *Guide to Stress Reduction.* Berkeley, Calif.: Celestial Arts, 1997.

Naparstek, B. *Staying Well with Guided Imagery.* New York: Warner, 1994.

Ornish, D. *Love and Survival: 8 Pathways to Intimacy and Health.* New York: Harper Perennial, 1998.

Rossman, M. *Guided Imagery for Self-Healing.* New York: H. J. Kramer/New World Library, 2000.

Schiffman, E. *Yoga: The Spirit and Practice of Moving into Stillness.* New York: Pocket Books, 1996.

Selye, H. *The Stress of Life.* New York: McGraw-Hill, 1956.

Tobias, M., and Stewart, M. *Stretch and Relax.* Los Angeles: Body Press, 1985.

Bibliography / References

Part I / Headaches, Stress, and the Nervous System

2. Understanding Your Headaches

The Biology of Migraine

Montagna, P. Molecular genetics of migraine headaches: a review. *Cephalalgia* 20 (2000): 3–14.

Evidence that part of the brain that controls head pain (referred to as the migraine generator) may be "burned out" as a result of repeated migraine attacks.

Welch, K. M. A., Nagesh, V., Aurora, S. K., and Gelman, N. Periaqueductal gray matter dysfunction in migraine: cause or burden of illness? *Headache* 41 (2001): 629–37.

A review of the genetics of migraine.

Sando, P. S., Ambrosini, A., Agosti, R. M., and Schoenen, J. Genetics of migraine: possible links to neurophysiological abnormalities. *Headache* 42 (2002): 365–77.

Comorbidities with Migraine

Ottman, R., and Lipton, R. B. Comorbidity of migraine and epilepsy. *Neurology* 44 (1994): 2105–10.

Lipton, R. B., Hamelsky, S. W., Kolodner, K. B., Steiner, T. J., and Stewart,

W. F. Migraine, quality of life, and depression: a population-based case-control study. *Neurology* 55 (5) (2000): 629–35.

The comorbidity of migraine with other disorders including mood disorders, epilepsy, stroke, and tremor.

Silberstein, S. D. Shared mechanisms and comorbidities in neurologic and psychiatric disorders. *Headache* 41 (suppl 1) (2001): 11–17.

Migraine in the Population

Lipton, R. B., Stewart, W. F., Diamond, S., Diamond, M., and Reed, M. L. Prevalence and burden of migraine in United States: results from the American migraine study II. *Headache* 41 (2001): 646–57.

Lipton, R. B., Stewart, W. F., and Simon, D. Medical consultation for migraine. Results from the American migraine study. *Headache* 38 (1998): 87–96.

Murray, C. J. L., and Lopez, A. D. Regional patterns of disability-free life expectancy and disability-adjusted life expectancy: global burden of disease study. *Lancet* 349 (1997): 1347–52.

This study examines the compromised mental, physical, and social functioning in migraine sufferers.

Terwindt, G. M., Ferrari, M. D., Tijhuis, M., Groenen, H. S. J., Picavet, H. S. J., and Launer, L. J. The impact of migraine on quality of life in the general population. The GEM study. *Neurology* 55 (5) (2000): 624–29.

A total of 688 migraine sufferers were interviewed regarding their treatment preferences and satisfaction with their migraine care.

Lipton, R. B., Stewart, W. F. Acute migraine therapy: do doctors understand what patients with migraine want from therapy? *Headache* 39 (suppl 2) (1999): S20–S26.

This survey showed prevalence of migraine is 17.2 percent in females, 6 percent males; that 31 percent of migraine sufferers had never seen a doctor for their headaches; 49 percent of migraine sufferers treated with over-the-counter medications only, 23 percent used prescription medication only, 23 percent used both, and 5 percent used no medication at all.

Lipton, R. B., Scher, A. I., Kolodner, K., Liberman, J., Steiner, T. J., and Stewart, W. F. Migraine in United States. Epidemiology and patterns of health care use. *Neurology* 58 (2002): 885–94.

A review of the disability caused by migraine. For example, about three-quarters of migraine sufferers have a reduced ability to function during attacks, with more than half reporting severe disability with the need for bed rest.

Holmes, W. F., MacGregor, E. A., and Dodick, D. Migraine-related disability. Impact and implications for sufferers' lives and clinical issues. *Neurology* 56 (suppl 1): (2001): S13–S19.

Migraine costs American employers about $13 billion per year because of missed work and impaired work function.

Hu, X. H., Markson, L. E., Lipton, R. B., Stewart, W. F., and Berger, M. L. Burden of migraine in United States. Disability and economic costs. *Archives of Internal Medicine* 159 (1999): 813–18.

Diagnosis of Migraine

International Headache Society. Classification and diagnostic criteria for headache disorders, cranial neuralgias and facial pain. *Cephalalgia* 8 (suppl 7) (1998): 1–96.

Cady, R. K., and Schreiber, C. P. Sinus headache or migraine? Considerations in making a differential diagnosis. *Neurology* 58 (suppl 6) (2002): S10–S14.

A discussion that migraine and tension headaches share a common basis.

Cady, R. K., Schreiber, C. P., Farmer, K., and Sheftell, F. Primary headaches: a convergence hypothesis. *Headache* 42 (2002): 204–16.

Evidence based on response to medication that the migraine spectrum goes from tension-type headache to full-blown migraine.

Lipton, R. B., Stewart, W. F., Cady, R., Hall, C., O'Quinn, S., Kuhn, T., and Gutterman, D. Sumatriptan for the range of headaches in migraine sufferers: results of the spectrum study. *Headache* 40 (2000): 783–91.

Daily Headache

Spierings, E. L. H. Chronic daily headache: a review. *Headache Quarterly* 11 (2000): 181–96.

Mathew, N. T., Reuveni, U., and Perez, F. Transformed or evolutive migraine. *Headache* 27 (1987): 102–6.

3. The Gift: Enhanced Responsiveness
of the Nervous System

Individuals with migraine respond differently to pain and pyschological stress.

Hassinger, H. J., Semenchuk, E. M., and O'Brien, W. H. Cardiovascular responses to pain and stress in migraine. *Headache* 39 (9) (1999): 605–15.

Evidence of brain hyperexcitability in migraine—the "enhanced responsiveness" of the nervous system.

Aurora, S. K., and Welch, K. M. A. Brain excitability in migraine: evidence from transcranial magnetic stimulation studies. *Current Opinions in Neurology* 11 (1988): 205–9.

Weiller, C., May, A., Limmroth, V., Juptner, M., Kaube, H., Schayck, R., Coenen, H. H., and Diener, H. C. Brainstem activation in spontaneous human migraine attacks. *Nature Medicine* 1 (1995): 658–60.

Welch, K. M. A., D'Andrea, G., Tepley, N., Barkley, G., and Ramadan, N. M. The concept of migraine as a state of central neuronal hyperexcitability. *Neurology Clinics* 8 (4) (1990): 817–28.

This study suggests that migraine sufferers have mild abnormalities in the balance between sympathetic and parasympathetic nervous system.

Mosek, A., Novak, V., Opfer-Gehrking, T. L., Swanson, J. W., and Low, P. A. Autonomic dysfunction in migraineurs. *Headache* 39 (1999): 108–17.

The visual part of the cerebral cortex is more excitable in migraine sufferers.

Aurora, S. K., Ahmad, B. K., Welch, K. M. A., Bhardhwaj, P., and Ramadan, N. M. Transcranial magnetic stimulation confirms hyperexcitability of occipital cortex in migraine. *Neurology* 50 (4) (1998): 1111–14.

Aurora, S. K., Cao, Y., Bowyer, S. M., and Welch, K. M. A. The occipital cortex is hyperexcitable in migraine: experimental evidence. *Headache* 39 (1999): 469–76.

4. Stress and the Nervous System and
5. Restoring Balance in the Nervous System

The groundbreaking initial article describing the three stages of the stress response.

Selye, H. A syndrome produced by diverse nocuous agents. *Nature* 138 (1936): 32.

Richter, C. P. On the phenomenon of sudden death in animals and man. *Psychosomatic Medicine* 19 (1957): 191–94.

This study describes the "3 Cs" of stress hardiness.

Kobasa, S. Stressful life events, personality, and health: an inquiry into hardiness. *Journal of Personality and Social Psychology* 37 (1979): 1–11.

Functional magnetic resonance imaging indicates that brain regions activated during meditation and relaxation have close links to control of the autonomic nervous system.

Lazar, S. W., Bush, G., Gollub, R. L., Fricchione, G. L., Khalsa, G., and Benson, H. Functional brain mapping of the relaxation response and meditation. *Neuroreport* 11 (7) (May 15, 2000): 1581–85.

Evidence that psychological stress (defined in a group of women taking care of demented relatives) resulted in delayed wound healing.

Kiecolt-Galser, J. K., Marucha, P. T., Malarkey, W. B., Mercado, A. M., and Glaser, R. Slowing of wound healing by psychological stress. *Lancet* 346 (1995): 1194–96.

Evidence that prolonged stress may produce volume loss in part of the brain called the hippocampus.

Sapolsky, R. M. Glucocorticoids and hippocampal atrophy in neuropsychiatric disorders. *Archives of general psychiatry* 57 (2000): 925–35.

Mental stress can cause constriction of coronary vessels.

Lacy, C. R., Contrada, R. J., Robbins, M. L., Tannenbaum, A. K., Moreyra, A. E., Chelton, S., and Kostis, J. B. Coronary vasoconstriction induced by mental stress (simulated public speaking). *American Journal of Cardiology* 75 (1995): 503–5.

A technical review of how our endocrine and nervous system responds to stress.

Chrousos, G. P., and Gold, P. W. The concepts of stress and stress system disorders. Overview of physical and behavioral homeostasis. *Journal of the American Medical Association* 267 (9) (1992): 1244–52.

An excellent review article on the adaptation response to stress and the concept of accumulating stress load that damages health.

McEwen, B. S. Protective and damaging effects of stress mediators. *New England Journal of Medicine* 338 (1998): 171–79.

The effect of social stress on baboons.

Sapolsky, R. Stress in the wild. *Scientific American* 262 (1990):116–23.

A pessimistic outlook (as evaluated from MMPI scores) correlates with higher mortality rate.

Maruta, T., Coligan, R. C., Malinchoc, M., and Offord, K. P. Optimists vs. pessimists: survival rate among medical patients over a 30-year period. *Mayo Clinic Proceedings* 75 (2000): 140–43.

One of several studies correlating stress with headache frequency.

Reynolds, D. J., and Hovanitz, C. A. Life events stress and headache frequency revisited. *Headache* 40 (2000): 111–18.

A study indicating that stress precedes onset of headache.

DeBenedittis, G., Lorenzetti, A., and Pieri, A. The role of stressful life events in the onset of chronic primary headache. *Pain* 41 (1990): 65–75.

Another study showing that migraine sufferers have a lower threshold to stress. The study also provides further evidence of the neuronal excitability of the migraine trait.

Rainero, I., Amanzioni, M., Vighetti, S., Bergamasco, B., Pinessi, L., and Benedetti, F. Quantitative EEG responses to ischaemic arm stress in migraine. *Cephalalgia* 21 (2001): 224–29.

One of several studies that show a correlation between headache and depression.

Silverstein, B., McKoy, E., Clauson, J., Perdue, L., and Raben, J. The correlation between depression and headache: the role played by generational changes in female achievement. *Journal of Applied Psychology* 25 (1995): 35–48.

An evaluation of why headaches tend to occur following transition from work to rest. Most individuals who experienced symptoms at times of leisure (such as weekends) show inability to relax and a high sense of work responsibility.

Vingerhoets, A. J., Van Huijgevoort, M., and Heck, G. L. Leisure sickness: a pilot study on its prevalence, phenomenology and background. *Psychotherapy and Psychosomatics* 71 (6) (2002): 311–17.

6. Taking Medication to Treat Your Headache

Summary of Drug Treatment

Diamond, S., Diamond, M., Silberstein, S., and Winner, P. Advances in migraine management: the roles of acute, prophylactic and rescue medications. *Headache Quarterly* 12 (2001): 183–94.

Tfelt-Hansen, P., and Welch, K. M. A. General principles of pharmacological treatment of migraine. In Olesen, J., Tfelt-Hansen, P., and Welch, K. M. A., eds. *The Headaches.* 2nd ed., 385–89. Philadelphia, Penn.: Lippincott Williams and Wilkins, 2000.

Medication Overuse Headache

An editorial on drug-induced rebound headache and medication overuse headache.

Silberstein, S. D., and Welch, K. M. A. Painkiller headache. *Neurology* 59 (2002): 972–74.

Different patterns of headache resulting from overuse of different headache-relieving medications.

Limmroth, V., Katsarava, Z., Fritsche, G., Przywara, S., and Diener, H. C. Features of medication overuse headache following overuse of different acute headache drugs. *Neurology* 59 (2002): 1011–14.

Part II / HARP: The Headache Reduction Program

7. Taking Control When Migraines Threaten

A review of cognitive-behavioral therapy of headache disorders. The combination of behavioral therapy with preventive medication results in a greater improvement than from either medication or cognitive-behavioral treatment alone.

Lake, A. E. Behavioral and nonpharmacologic treatments of headache. *Medical Clinics of North America* 8 (4) (July 2001): 1055–75.

A meta-analysis of studies indicate that behavioral interventions result in approximately 35 to 50 percent reduction in migraine and tension-type headaches.

Penzien, D. B., Rains, J. C., and Andrasik, F. Behavioral management of recurrent headache: three decades of experience and empiricism. *Applied Psychophysiology Biofeedback* 27 (2002): 163–81.

Burns, D. *The Feeling Good Handbook.* New York: Plume, 1989.

Passchier, J., Mourik, J., Brienen, J. A., and Hunfeld, J. A. M. Cognitions, emotions, and behavior of patients with migraine when taking medication during an attack. *Headache* 38 (6) (1998): 458–64.

8. Natural Ways to Prevent Headaches

Anderson, B. *Stretching at Your Computer or Desk.* Bolinas, Calif.: Shelter Publications, 1997.

Benson, H. *The Relaxation Response.* New York: William Morrow, 1975.

Hanh, T. N. *Peace Is Every Step: The Path of Mindfulness in Everyday Life.* New York: Bantam Books, 1976.

9. Self-Care for Well-Being: Beyond Headache Reduction

This book is required reading for HARP participants. It also cites the research done by Kobasa, and Greiff's Five Ls of Success.

Benson, H., and Stewart, E. M. *The Wellness Book: The Comprehensive Guide to Maintaining Health and Treating Stress-Related Illness.* New York: Simon & Schuster, 1992.

Fox, J. *Poetic Medicine.* New York: Tarcher/Putnam, 1997.

Cousins, N. *Anatomy of an Illness as Perceived by the Patient.* New York: Bantam Books, 1981.

Kobasa, S. Stressful life events, personality, and health: an inquiry into hardiness. *Journal of Personality and Social Psychology* 37 (1979): 1–11.

Guided imagery is a relaxation technique based on visualizing positive image and body awareness. Use of these techniques by chronic headache sufferers resulted a significant improvement not only in headache but in vitality and mental health.

Mannix, L. K., Chandurkar, R. S., Rybicki, R. S., Tusek, L. A., and Solomon, G. D. Effect of guided imagery on quality of life for patients with chronic tension-type headache. *Headache* 39 (1999): 326–34.

Naparstek, B. *Staying Well with Guided Imagery.* New York: Warner, 1994.

Ornish, D. *Love and Survival: 8 Pathways to Intimacy and Health.* New York: Harper Perennial, 1998.

Index

In this index, *f* indicates figure and *b* indicates box.

About the Authors

IAN LIVINGSTONE, M.D., a board-certified neurologist, is medical director of the Princeton Headache Clinic. *The Castle Connolly Guide* lists him as one of the top doctors in the New York metropolitan area.

DONNA NOVAK, R.N., is a board-certified nurse practitioner in women's health and a cofounder of the Princeton Headache Clinic. Novak is currently an editorial director for *Nursing Spectrum* magazine.